SLEEP

How to Sleep Like a Baby Even if You Have Sleep Apnea!

(Get Rid of Sleep Apnea for Good With Simple Natural Exercises)

Terri Holmes

Published by Tomas Edwards

© **Terri Holmes**

All Rights Reserved

Sleep: How to Sleep Like a Baby Even if You Have Sleep Apnea! (Get Rid of Sleep Apnea for Good With Simple Natural Exercises)

ISBN 978-1-990268-40-3

Legal & Disclaimer

The information contained in this book is not designed to replace or take the place of any form of medicine or professional medical advice. The information in this book has been provided for educational and entertainment purposes only.

The information contained in this book has been compiled from sources deemed reliable, and it is accurate to the best of the Author's knowledge; however, the Author cannot guarantee its accuracy and validity and cannot be held liable for any errors or omissions. Changes are periodically made to this book. You must consult your doctor or get professional medical advice before using any of the suggested remedies, techniques, or information in this book.

Upon using the information contained in this book, you agree to hold harmless the Author from and against any damages, costs, and expenses, including any legal fees potentially resulting from the application of any of the information provided by this guide. This disclaimer applies to any damages or injury caused by the use and application, whether directly or indirectly, of any advice or information presented, whether for breach of contract, tort, negligence, personal injury, criminal intent, or under any other cause of action.

You agree to accept all risks of using the information presented inside this book. You need to consult a professional medical practitioner in order to ensure you are both able and healthy enough to participate in this program.

Table of Contents

Introduction

This book contains proven steps and strategies on how to manage and treat your sleep apnea.

This book will allow you to understand what sleep apnea is, what its effects are, the changes that you can make in your lifestyle to avoid it, and the treatment you can undergo so that you will be able to finally have a good night's sleep. This book also includes the outcomes that you can expect after the treatment.

With the information that you will get in this book, you will be able to take control of the way you sleep so you can wake up feeling refreshed and ready to tackle on the challenges you face every day.You do not have to feel hopeless about your condition.As you will learn in this book, the cure is in your hands.You can free yourself from your sleep troubles and live a fulfilling life.Read on and find out how.

Thanks again for downloading this book, I hope you enjoy it!

Chapter 1 What You Eat Helps A Lot

The quantity of sleep is just as important as the quality of sleep, and believe it or not, the food and drink you enjoy has effects on both the quantity and quality of your sleep.

Whatever you eat at dinner time has a huge impact on whether you'll get a good night's sleep or not, because dinner is the last "job" your digestive system has to do before it stops working for the night.So, it is important to make sure that what you put in your digestive system at dinner time is not only easy to process, but foods that promote sleep and increase the quality of your sleep.

For example, eating food rich in omega-3 oils have been found to increase the quality of sleep because omega-3 reduces anxiety and even depression.It also improves insulin production and helps muscles grow, while it gives the nutrients the brain needs to repair itself.Again, all repairs to the body are done at night, so eating something that will help your body do all those repairs properly will certainly boost the performance of your body and mind the next day.

Best sources for omega-3 are low-mercury fish like tuna and other seafood.You can also take food supplements of omega-3 and it will work just fine.Make sure to have your fill of your omega-3 at least 2 – 3 hours before bedtime for best results.

You can also benefit from taking MCT (Medium-chain triglycerides) oils at night before going to sleep.MCT oils helps burn body fat while you sleep, and is immediately used by your brain because it is converted into ketones once it enters your system.Of course, if you're not used to taking this oil, start slow, like 1 teaspoon and work your way up to a maximum of 2 tablespoons a night.

You can also try herbal teas that induce sleep.Chamomile is a known relaxant and can help you de-stress so you can fall asleep faster.Warm milk and oatmeal have also been found to be good for people who have trouble sleeping.Of course, food and drinks with caffeine and sugar should be avoided as these foods actually inhibit sleep.

Alcohol works for some people, but try not to make it a habit.When you drink alcohol all the time, your tolerance for alcohol will go higher, making it impossible for you to sleep until you've maxed it out.So, try to pull yourself away after two glasses of wine or two bottles of beer.

Toxins also prevent sleep, so you need to pack up onantioxidants so your body can get rid of the toxins.So, focus your diet on high nutrient fruits and vegetables, and drink herbal tea at night and maybe green tea during the day.

Virgin coconut oil is also an effective sleep agent.Virgin coconut oil helps our body manufacture more sleep hormones.You can take about 1 -2 tablespoons of virgin coconut oil in the morning and at bedtime.

It is also highly recommended that you stop eating at least 4 hours before you sleep.This gives your digestive system enough time to finish all the work it needs to do with the dinner you have just had before it closes shop.It is also a good idea not to eat hard-to-digest proteins at night as this would keep your digestive system busy, which, in turn, will keep you awake.

Going back to foods that don't work if you want to get good sleep, it is important to mention that some foods have different effects on different people.For example, grains and other refined carbs tend to push sugars to go zap and then die down almost as quickly. This causes more stress to the body, further impeding sleep.

It has also been discovered lately that many people have a magnesium deficiency, and this also leads to other bodily functions not working properly.Adding magnesium to your body (as a food supplement) before you sleep increases the quality of your sleep.

Now, while all these foods encourage sleep, try not to eat too much.Just enough, consumed regularly, will do the trick.

Chapter 2: Different Types Of Sleep Apnea

There are three types of Sleep Apnea:

Obstructive Sleep Apnea

Central Sleep Apnea

Complex Sleep Apnea

Out of these three, the OSA or Obstructive Sleep Apnea is the most common type, and it is also diagnosed instantly.

Let's take it a bit further and understand them separately.

Obstructive Sleep Apnea (OSA)

We have already discussed a bit of OSA above. The name Obstructive is enough to indicate that due to an obstruction, the person is not able to breathe well. But there is something more intricate and complex that goes on inside the body during the time OSA strikes.

Obstructive Sleep Apnea is majorly related to body functioning. Basically, several body parts are connected with it. From your throat to the chest and diaphragm, those body parts which have a direct link with the respiratory system are somewhat affected. Also, problems in these body parts can become a cause for Sleep Apnea.

OSA has a separate measurement index, called the Apnea-Hypopnea index (AHI). It is through this index that the doctors can readily analyze the intensity of this disease and provide the methods to cure it.

To give you a brief idea about the AHI, this is simply a measurement to know how many episodes does a person has in an hour. It is formulated after several episodes of apneas added with the number of Hypopnea, averaged for an hour.

Understanding the difference between Apnea and Hypopnea:

Where apnea means that there will be no breathing for a short amount of time, Hypopnea implies that there will be shallow breathing. In Hypopnea the airway is not entirely blocked, or you can say that it is partially blocked.

Both Apnea and Hypopnea are observed in Obstructive Sleep Apnea. Rest everything remains the same. Like, how the brain is forced to wake up in the middle of your sleep and instruct the airways to open up again.

As per the AHI, there are further three types of OSA:

Mild OSA: This type has an AHI index of 5-15. Until and unless, the number of Sleep Apnea episodes is limited within this range, there is no need to worry much. A mild OSA can be treated with ease and with minimal efforts.

Moderate OSA: The AHI for this type of OSA ranges between 15 to 30. Now, this is where you need to worry a bit. 15 to 30 episodes of apnea or Hypopnea is a bit much. The person who is suffering from it needs medical attention.

Severe OSA: This is where things get pretty serious; here the AHI increases above 30. This means that a person has more than 30 breaks in the normal breathing cycle in an hour.

OSA is a simple form of Sleep Apnea, but it can be a bit dangerous if not treated or addressed on time. Because with OSA, the muscles that are contracting and blocking the airway may continue to deteriorate.

Now, the ball is in your park to get your OSA diagnosed on time. Because if it goes unchecked, there are a lot of other problems that can show up due to it. To name a few, high blood pressure, cardiovascular diseases, stroke, falling asleep while driving, diabetes or even depression.

The reason for the risk of developing all these conditions is due to the complex interconnectedness of our body. As every significant part of our body has a direct or an indirect link with each other, an anomaly in one part can bring about a ripple effect in others.

Central Sleep Apnea

Central Sleep Apnea (CSA) is a bit different from Obstructive Sleep Apnea. In CSA, the issue is with how the brain functions and not with the throat.

The difference lies in not whether you can breathe or not, but it is with the fact that the brain does not give a command to the muscles to breathe. And that is why it is called Central Sleep Apnea because the issue stems from the inability of the brain's normal functioning.

The lower brainstem is responsible for breathing. And in CSA, the individual's lower brainstem is affected, which causes Sleep Apnea. So in a sense, this is what brings about a significant difference in the working and incidence of Central Sleep Apnea.

CSA is a rarer form of Sleep Apnea. And it occurs in on and off cycles. And most of the time, the primary area of concern is the brain. But there have been cases where the heart is also responsible for this condition.

What happens in CSA?

When I say the brain, it means that the Central Nervous System has a significant role in CSA. Usually, the brain gives instructions to the diaphragm to take a breath.

But in CSA, the brain forgets or is unable to do so. Without the diaphragm initiating a breath, the respiratory cycle won't complete. There is no inhalation of air, which means that the amount of oxygen will start to decrease. Consequently, the amount of carbon dioxide will begin to increase.

Once that happens, the brain won't get enough oxygen and it kind of resets after knowing that what's going on in the body. Another dimension of difference between CSA and OSA lies among the causes that result in the onslaught of such conditions.

But, the essential thing to understand is that most of the time, the causes for OSA are known and are quite visible. With CSA, these causes are not very visible. There can be many reasons as to why someone is suffering from CSA.

So, I guess you get the picture. CSA is a kind of involuntary breathing, where a person's breath is not even under their control because the part which is responsible for breathing does not function properly.

Types of CSA

Several kinds of CSA have been recorded and observed until now. Some of them are induced by a health condition, while for others, the cause is not known.

-**Primary Central Sleep Apnea:** Until now, the cause of this kind of Sleep Apnea is not known. But how breathing continues is a bit distinct. In this case, two things are worth mentioning. One is the breathing effort, and the other is the airflow.

-**Cheyne-Stokes Breathing Pattern:** Problems like a heart condition, stroke, or even kidney failure can give birth to this kind of CSA. The breathing pattern is in rhythm rather than in a pattern with this kind of CSA.

-**High Altitude Periodic Breathing:** When you are sleeping at altitudes higher than 15000 feet, this kind of Sleep Apnea can be observed. Although the pattern of breathing is similar to the Cheyne Stokes, the factors which cause it are different.

-**Drug Abuse:** Drug or substance abuse, especially of the opioid category, can also lead to the development of CSA. Here, the breathing pattern is not fixed. It may fluctuate or can even stop abruptly. Also, some people may experience breathing issues associated with OSA.

Complex Sleep Apnea: A Disease or Not?

Well, the debate is still ongoing. Complex Sleep Apnea is a rather new kind of Sleep Apnea, and there is no consensus among the scientific community about its origin. But as we are on the topic, why not discuss it too.

So, in definition, Complex Sleep Apnea is a mix of obstructive and central Sleep Apnea. More specifically, this type of Sleep Apnea is also referred to as Complex Sleep

Apnea Syndrome or CompSAS. In this, a person experiences more than 5 episodes of CSA in less than an hour.

Added to it, these episodes of breathing issues persist after there have been cases of Obstructive Sleep Apnea. There have been reports of such a condition occurring when the patients are regularly using the CPAP device for their Apnea treatment.

I know this is all a bit confusing. But that is the major problem around it. In some cases, there is a specific reason, and in others, the causative factors are interrelated with each other. Somewhere the CSA is responsible for such an issue and in others the problems caused due to CSA become the cause for CompSAS.

Chapter 3: Mind, Body And Spirit: An Act Of Reconnection

For centuries, holistic healers have been largely ignored when they have tried to explain how the connection between the mind, body and spirit works. It has just been recently that modern science and researchers have caught up.There have been some significant discoveries including some connections to how well people deal with or even manage to recover from serious diseases including cancer and heart disease. In one study, researchers at the University of California at San Francisco (1) discovered that breast cancer patients who participated in weekly group therapy sessions were able to survive as much as two times longer than those who did not. In another study researchers at the University of California at Los Angeles found that people facing melanoma surgery benefitted greatly from receiving education about reducing stress levels, coping skills plus counseling each week. Those patients who were given these skills had a fifty percent lower risk of recurrence and were thirty times less likely to die from their disease.

For the last ten years, researchers from various universities the world over have looked at how the mind, body and spirit work together. There have been studies that show the benefit of prayer or even just quiet meditation for those who do not follow a particular faith at times of a health crisis. But, you don't have to be facing the dangers of a serious disease like cancer to get the benefits of reconnecting. You do not have to do anything "weird" or anything that you are not comfortable with either. Remember, the goal here is to reestablish a balance, not to create a worse one.

Before going further, here are a few key points that are important to keep in mind:

I am not advocating one type of religion over another. In fact, you don't have to follow a religion at all for this reconnection. People without religious faith, even atheists can have a spiritual connection that does not tie into a deity at all.

If you are not comfortable with any suggestion that is offered in this book, please feel free to skip it, modify it or find an alternative that does work for you.

There is no single suggestion that will work for everyone so keep that in mind as well.

In Chapter One, I briefly mentioned what happens after a night of less than restful or interrupted sleep. We feel groggy or cranky. We might forget little details. We might even do strange things like put the car keys in the freezer or put the butter in the dryer while we are rushing to do the laundry. These are all frustrating little things but have you ever stopped to consider how these things happen in the first place?

We separate the mind, the body and the spirit into three parts and then assign them each tasks. We expect the brain to help us remember things, to know how to do certain tasks and to be able to learn how to do others. We expect the brain to keep us from putting our car keys in the freezer because it knows that they do not belong there and yet, here are our icy cold keys once again.

We expect our body to do the physical things during the day, of course. We don't remember back to our basic science classes where we learned that every movement is directed by the brain thanks to the extensive nerve network. We treat the body like a machine at times but then forget that even machines must be recharged in some way so that they can work properly.

And from our spirit, we expect the ability to calm us, to nurture us and to restore us in times of great stress. But, again, we forget that we must consciously tap into that spirit for the connection to even be there.

If the body is not rested, it can get injured but even more deeply, it means the mind did not get a chance to recharge either. If you are exhausted mentally and physically there is no way to tap into your spiritual side. See how they are all connected to one another?Being upset can keep you from sleeping. Being sick or injured can keep you from sleeping. Being stressed or worried can keep you from sleeping. But, nurturing yourself, mind, body and spirit can restore your health, your mental clarity and your spiritual side once again.

Chapter 4: Diagnosing Sleep Apnea

Diagnosing the condition may be tricky, because more often than not people dismiss this as a mere snoring habit. If you are one of those who have symptoms that are mentioned above, then you should try to have them diagnosed. Here are some common methods to diagnose Sleep Apnea.

Polysomnogram

Polysomnogram (PSG) is a sleep study conducted for detecting Sleep Apnea. It involves monitoring brain activity, heart beats, eye motions and the blood pressure of the patient. The oxygen levels in your blood can also be detected using this technique. The patient's chest motions can indicate whether he is breathing easily or not. If it is observed that the patient requires extra efforts to breathe normally, then it may be a case of Sleep Apnea. Many times the doctors also conduct a "split-night" study, wherein a CPAP machine is used during the second half of the study for detection.

Portable Monitors

A portable monitor comes in handy to check whether you have Sleep Apnea or not. This monitor is very popular due to its user-friendly operation and compact size. The monitor helps in documenting similar kind of data provided by PSG technique, without having to go to a clinic to get the test done. This portable, home-based monitor can detect the following things:

a) Oxygen levels in the blood

b) Heart beat rate

c)Airflow movement across the nose while breathing

d)Easy or difficult chest movements

Sleep Studies

Sleep studies refer to an in-depth study of the patient's sleeping patterns. It indicates whether the patient gets sound sleep or it is often disrupted with the patient waking up frequently. Through this study, it becomes easier to understand the real cause of the patient's disruptive sleep pattern. The doctor also needs to study how severe the sleep disorder is and to prescribe an appropriate line of medication.

Physical Examination

A physical examination is a must in order to diagnose Sleep Apnea problems in children, since they show prominent physical signs of this disorder. Enlarged tonsils can easily be identified through a physical examination, wherein the doctor may check the mouth, nose or tonsils of the patient.

A lot of times, you may suspect that you are suffering from insomnia, when it could turn out to be sleep apnea. You may confuse the symptoms of other conditions or disorders and may eventually pass it off as a common problem.

Let's make a list of some important questions, you can ask yourself to determine the exact case of you sleeplessness or excessive sleepiness.

Quiz to determine whether you are suffering from Sleep Apnea

1) Do you snore everyday or at least 3 nights in a week?

a) Yes

b) No

2) Does your snoring disrupt other people's sleep?

a) Yes

b) No

3)Are you facing at least 3 of the above mentioned sleep apnea symptoms?

a) Yes

b) No

4) Have you developed a sudden habit of sleeping during daytime?

a) Yes

b)No

5) Is your collar size relatively bigger than others?

a) Yes

b) No

The above questions will help you analyze if your snoring problems are indeed due to Sleep Apnea. If you find yourself answering yes more often than not, then there is a good chance that you are suffering from Sleep Apnea and need to consult a doctor immediately.

Chapter 5: Types Of Sleep & Sleep Cycles

You might be thinking "what a ridiculous title for a chapter – surely you are asleep or you are not". Well not so. There have been many studies done on how human beings sleep, and it has been found to be a more complex science than might appear at first. Rather than any sense that when we close our eyes and go to sleep, we move into a block of deep sleep, rather it has been found that we move through a series of sleep rhythms, with associated movements, all of which are fundamental to waking up in the morning refreshed or not. It is important to get at least a degree of understanding of these if you are having problems with sleep – whether that is getting to sleep in the first place, waking through the night, or something else. In the remainder of this chapter we explore these different phases and rhythms of sleep.

Circadian Rhythm – Our Body Clock

To fully understand how we sleep, when we feel tired and so on, we need to understand a little about why we feel tired at certain times at all. Most living organisms have in-built, and usually subconscious, reaction to their external processes and environment. At a basic level this means that changes take place directly related to the rhythms of a day – typically when it is light and when it is dark though of course that is subject to variation. Ask yourself why it is that most activity across the natural world takes place when it is daylight. The birds chirp when the sun is coming up (or somehow they know it is coming up) and then chirp again as the sun goes down, before they settle down to roost. Humans, of course, are part of that natural world too, and they also typically follow natural patterns associated with the sun and daylight – albeit that for much of the human population there is the capacity to alter how long it can stay light and dark.

For human beings, then, these essential rhythms take place over the 24 hour cycle, and this wider phenomenon is known as the Circadian Clock. Effectively light and dark are the primary drivers for when we feel awake and when we feel tired, though of course these are not the only things which affect our mindset. You might feel more tired after exercise, a hard day at work and so on, but underpinning this is the overall natural sleep cycle associated with our environment which affects all of us. We have talked a little about shift working already – in effect such ways of working can have to drive against our natural rhythms, and it can be this which can make shift work have particular effects – in addition you are likely to be having to sleep when it is light – going against natural instincts. It is important to try and make sure there are not too many unnatural influences on your own body clock – we will discuss this a little later.

Phases of sleep

Now that you have an understanding of your own tiredness, sleeping rhythms, and the underlying phenomenon of the Circadian Clock we can explore the different phases of sleep. This brings us back to previous comments pertaining to the fact that all sleep is not the same – if you think about it, this can explain why, for example, you may have been in bed all night, but still wake up tired – it is possible you may not have had the appropriate amount of the type of sleep you need to feel fully refreshed. Let us explore the different types of sleep, and see if you can identify what might be happening when you go to sleep.

When you first fall asleep, you will enter what is known as a period of non-rapid eye movement (NREM) sleep. Studies have shown that this phase of sleep has three separate stages, each of which sees you fall more deeply asleep, that is it is harder for you to be roused (and it may be a little confusing if you are woken up at this point). Normally, the next, and fourth stage of sleep you will enter will be what is known as rapid eye movement sleep (or REM). This is typically the stage of sleep that people have heard of most – at this point you will have come out of deeper sleep, and may be on the verge of wakefulness. It is at this point that you will find that you are dreaming. According to the Sleep Council, each of these cycles of four stages lasts about 90 minutes and a good night's sleep will see five or six cycles which should include all stages I order for you to be fully rested. If you have a disturbed night's sleep, or do not go to bed for long enough then you will not feel rested – this si why it is important to try and get the requisite amount of hours of sleep you need – we will consider this next.

How much sleep do I need?

All this talk of phases, cycles and stages of sleep makes it sound as if there is a lot going on when we sleep! Sometimes there is, but the critical thing is to make sure that you manage to allow yourself the space to have the appropriate hours of sleep to best fit you. How much sleep you need will depend on a number of factors, but one of the critical issues is what age you are. The following are recommended amounts of sleep.

For a newborn baby, up to three months old, around fourteen to seventeen hours is recommended, though it may be that slightly higher or lower could also be appropriate – invariably, in the very early days a baby will wake and sleep in shorter bursts as it adjusts to the Circadian Clock we discussed earlier. As a baby gets older, between four and eleven months, then the requirement for sleep drops a little, to between twelve and fifteen hours, but again with some latitude above and below this figure.

As a child learns to walk and move around, over the ages of one and two, then the core requirement falls again to between eleven and fourteen hours. Note though that these are very slight and gradual changes. By the time a child is one or two years old they will likely be having one or two naps during the day as well as their longer night-time sleep – though of course this will vary from child to child. By pre-school age, from three to five years, the core hours are around ten to thirteen hours. Changes are likely to be less apparent between the ages of about six and thirteen, with the core hours likely to be between nine and eleven hours, though again with an appropriate option either up or down. Teenagers should require less sleep again, though you may well find that not to be the case, or that sleep patterns are very different – often this can be for hormonal reasons. Adults, of whatever age generally require at least seven hours of sleep, and up to nine hours - again some will need a little more, some a little less, and by over the age of sixty-five, it is expected that someone will still require at least seven hours sleep but may be able to do with I a little less than younger adults.

Of course this is just an outline, and what will suit one person of one age will not necessarily suit another. This is why it is important to be aware of your own needs and do what you can to achieve your sleep goals.

Chapter 6: Mild Bouts Of Sleep Apnea

According to major sleep apnea studies, gender, weight, age, genetics and race are factors that can contribute to the risk of developing this complication. Alcohol and smoking can also put you at risk or worsen and exiting condition.

On the other hand, smokers are 2.5 times more likely to have sleep apnea because smoking causes the airway tissues to swell. As a result, the air passage is constricted, contributing to sleep apnea.

During treatment, patients are advised to make lifestyle changes, which includes quitting smoking and reducing alcohol consumption. In fact, quitting the habit is essential in the successful treatment of apnea smokers.

With this said, below are some of the simple things you can do on your own to overcome or at least relieve some of the symptoms of Sleep Apnea.

Lose Weight

Obesity increases the risk of sleep apnea. This happens especially to those diagnosed with OSA. Unlike CSA, OSA is a function of mass in the air passages. If a person is sufficiently overweight, some of the mass that is built up in the body is located along the airways. In certain postures that mass can exert pressure on the passages causing those passages to close. The closure triggers a nervous response that alerts the body to wake up and readjust the position, or begin breathing via the mouth.

By losing just a small percentage of weight, one can help significantly with reduction in the case of OSA. Several studies have proven weight loss to be a first line defense in reducing the symptoms of OSA.

Limit Alcohol and Smoking

Tobacco and alcohol have dire consequences and can worsen sleep apnea by aggravating its symptoms, including increased breathing pauses and more labored snoring. Quitting both vices are the best option for someone diagnosed with OSA. For CSA, there is no direct link, but the alcohol and tobacco can result in OSA and that will complicate the person who is already suffering from CSA.

If you must drink, avoid alcohol at night or at least 6 hours before you get to bed.

Alcohol relaxes the muscles located at the back of the throat, and this causes an obstruction.

In addition to alcohol, caffeinated drinks, sedatives such as sleeping pills and anti allergy medication can have an effect on apnea.

Diet

From a holistic point of view, it is best for those diagnosed with sleep apnea, to fast at least once a week, if your health permits. It is also important that you have a good balance of iron and vitamin C in your diet. Reduce the amount of soy products in your diet and reduce dairy as well.Both of these food groups have negative side effects in oxygen exchange in the blood.

Studies also show that sleep apneics are more likely those who engage in unhealthy eating habits. Because apneics are typically sleep deprived, they are likely to have increased cravings specifically for carbohydrates, fat, protein and saturated fatty acids. In which case, they are also at more risk of gaining weight. This starts a vicious cycle. To stop this cycle, practice self-discipline and plan diets carefully. As much as possible, stick to healthy foods and eat moderately.

Keep Your Nasal Passages Open

Nasal allergies can further complicate the disorder. And it will make getting sleep much more difficult. When such allergies are out of control, a sleep apneic will have much more trouble breathing.It that can be dangerous, especially in the case of Obstructive Sleep Apnea. Items such as saline sprays, nasal dilators, and breathing strips could help in this regard.

Keep a steady Sleeping Schedule

One of the most crucial steps in dealing with sleep apnea is to arrange a sleeping schedule and sticking to it. Ensuring that you receive enough sleep every night is essential. A steady sleep schedule may be able to help relieve or reduce the episodes.

Chapter 7: Sleep Supplements

The following sleep supplements are best combined with a willingness to try new techniques and methods that can help maximize the quality of sleep.

Many people have trouble getting to sleep because of bad habits such as smoking, worrying, drinking, etc. Some natural sleep supplements can interfere with medication you may already be taking. Even herbal teas and natural melatonin tablets may have side effects.

Never take anything in combination with anti-depressants or other medication without consulting your doctor first. Pregnant women should be especially careful about what medicines they put into their bodies as well.

One third of all adults will suffer from sleep deprivation at some stage in their life, even if you don't feel like your problems are major, it's a good idea to get into a good sleep routine. Knowing the right holistic medicines will help immensely, because it prevents the need to rely on sleeping pills.

Ginkgo   Biloba

The history of Gingko Biloba has its origins in Eastern China. It has since been distributed and marketed as a sleep supplement throughout the word. Since 2800 BC, Chinese medical techniques have made extensive use of the Maindenhair tree which grows Ginkgo Biloba.

They have found it to be a major therapeutic aid in traditional medicine, and found that the roots, fruits and leaves from this tree are particularly useful. They can treat asthma, anxiety and other disorders and illnesses.

Since the 1960's western nations have made subcomponents of the plant commercially available, and marketed it as a health supplement. Consumers must do their research to find natural or organic versions of this supplement, and not buy a cheaper uncertified supplement that hasn't gone through extensive quality and purity tests. Some of the lesser quality supplements end up containing buckwheat, or rutin which is not helpful as a sleep aid. A 2001 pilot study published in Pharmacopsychiatry revealed that people who have depression had their symptoms reduced by Gingko Biloba, and also had their insomnia treated. One only needs to take 250mg to see positive results. The plant works by reducing symptoms of anxiety, fatigue and stress, which in turn enhances relaxation and improves sleep quality. Taking it half an hour or an hour before bed produces the best results. Gingko Biloba also allows for REM sleep to occur. According to Holland and Barratt, the herb extract also boosts cognitive functions such as attention, memory, and mental processing speed, especially in adults who may have Alzheimer's.

Magnesium

There are varying ways to take this sleep supplement; some people find it easier to take in the morning with breakfast, while some take it in the evening. The best way to find out the most effective time for you is by trying it at different times of the day and on different days. It's not uncommon for some people, especially women, to suffer from low magnesium levels. Healthy magnesium levels promote better sleep and can even assist with a quicker metabolism. Magnesium also contributes to the health of your bones and heart. We receive magnesium from leafy, dark greens, chocolate, coffee, and many other sources. Older adults are particularly at risk of having low magnesium levels, and may benefit from supplements. Magnesium also plays a crucial role in the production of energy, activating ATP, which is fuel for the cells in the body. Magnesium also regulates blood pressure, which in turn makes it easier to get to sleep.

People with low magnesium levels often report that they wake often in the night, due to low neurotransmitters that help transmit sleep. Magnesium also helps the restless-leg syndrome sleep disorder. Magnesium regulates the body's stress system and reduces levels of anxiety too. Lower levels of anxiety can in turn promote better gut health and a longer night's sleep without waking up.

Valerian   Root

Valerian root; the official name is valerian officinalis. It's an herb commonly found in Asia, North America, and Europe. Its earthy smell is partly responsible for its sedative effects and distinct taste. It is available in liquid form (people even drink it as a tea), or as a capsule. Strangely enough, most researchers are unsure of exactly how it works. They believe that it increases the same chemicals and neurotransmitters that magnesium does, but especially GABA (gamma aminobutyric acid), which results in a calming effect on the entire body. As mentioned before, valerian root should not be taken by everyone because it is a strong herb. Pregnant women especially, and toddlers, should not take it without consulting their doctor first. It should not be combined with other sedative drugs, as the effect on the body could cause addiction. The best time to take valerian root is right before bedtime because it causes instant drowsiness. It is never a good idea to take it before driving or operating heavy machinery, and especially in the morning.

Glycine

What is glycine? The name glycine originates from the Greek word for sweet. Glycine is an amino acid that creates proteins within the body, maintaining the tissue and creating essential substances. It is something that the body naturally produces, but it can be found in a dietary supplement or foods rich in protein. Glycine has many health benefits, such as being able to make glutathione, which is a powerful antioxidant. Glutathione helps prevent cells from becoming damaged, which can in turn stop diseases from occurring because exposure is limited. Without enough glycine, bodies produce less glutathione, which negatively affects how the body handles oxidative stress. Over time, this can become a real problem for fitness levels.

Glycine is readily available as a powder and can be added to drinks and food very easily. It can also be added to coffee, tea, soup, yogurt, protein shakes and more. Supplementing glycine is incredibly safe, as long as the dosage is appropriate. Studies have shown fitness gurus use up to 90 grams of the powder a day, without any serious side effects (although this is not recommended). Glycine is the vital amino acid used in collagen, which is the main structure for tissue that connects bone, skin, ligaments and cartilage. It can be found in varying dosages in meat, but a less commonly known fact is that it can also be found in gelatin. This is a substance made from collagen, and it is added to various foods to improve the consistency of certain foods. Glycine can also preserve muscle mass providing effective treatment for cancer patients or burn victims. More research is however being conducted to learn more about this amino acid. Glycine may reduce muscle depletion, malnutrition and other conditions where the body is under stress. There are many benefits of Glycine, but the main reason to take it is if you have trouble getting to or staying asleep. While there are several other supplements to take as listed in this book, this particular amino acid lowers the core body temperature (as mentioned earlier, this can be a factor in preventing a good night's sleep).

Many people have taken glycine and reported that it takes less time to fall asleep, and even increases sleep quality! It also has the added effect of improving cognitive skills, much like many other supplements.

Glycine may be an incredible alternative to a market that is over-saturated with sleeping pills that only cause drowsiness during the day anyway.

Lavender

Lavender is especially helpful and recommended by sleep experts because of its qualities that reduce anxiety. It is an anxiolytic. It reduces uncomfortable feelings such as anger, agitation and irritation. It is also a suitable pain reliever.

It works by improving sleep quality and has lavender which causes deep, slow-wave sleep. It can aid sleep quality as much as a low dosage of the sedative lorazepam. It can be both swallowed and inhaled.

L-Theanine

There's much evidence that proves this amino acid (found in tea leaves) enhances sleep quality. Some sleep doctors regularly encourage their patients to consume tea because it has less caffeine than coffee. Furthermore, decaffeinated tea can add to a ritual before bed that relaxes the body.

Think of it like powering down at night. Even in the morning, drinking a cup of herbal tea is refreshing, and soothes the mind and body, but if you really don't like hot drinks, L-Theanine can be found in the form of a supplement. Not only is it beneficial for soothing the body before bed time, it also centers you spiritually and helps with focusing on tasks at hand.

In the late 1940's, scientists in Japan discovered L-Theanine in tea and in mushrooms. It is thought to add a broth like taste, which comes from Unami. Unami helps power up a faster metabolism, and also contributes to the feeling of being 'full' after a meal. This in turn lengthens the amount of time in between meals. It has many rewards and health benefits. L-Theanine also boosts neurotransmitters that regulate emotion and the state of being alert. Many cognitive skills are also enhanced, which in turn promotes relaxation. If you are drinking too much coffee, decaffeinated tea may be an alternative because sometimes reaching for a hot drink can be as much about habit as anything else. L-Theanine also releases chemicals that promote feelings of calm, as well as protecting the mind against anxiety. It enhances natural brain waves that indicate being relaxed while awake. If you have experienced being in the creative state of 'flow', meditating or daydreaming, these are the alpha brain waves at work that enhance the same ability to relax. Another good reason to take L-Theanine is that it is not a sedative, so the drowsiness that occurs with some medication won't take place the following morning. Furthermore, it has been linked to sleep improvements in those with ADHD and other disorders.

Chapter 8: The Facts And Myths Of Sleep And Sleep Deprivation

There are a lot of myths and fallacies concerning sleep. These misconceptions can give a misleading view of how a person perceives the concept of sleep and sleeping. These can be possibly taken as truths that might adversely affect behaviors and attitudes concerning sleep.

Myth 1: Functioning during the daytime is not affected by a mere one hour less of sleep in a night.

The Facts: Losing even one hour of sleep from the recommended time can and will affect a person's ability to think properly and respond quickly to stimuli.

Myth 2: The body is able to adjust to numerous sleep schedules.

The Facts: It can take up to one week or more for the body to adjust to time zones and night shift work schedules.

Myth 3: Extra night time sleep can treat excessive fatigue during the day time.

The Facts: The quality of sleep can affect daytime functioning even more so than the amount of time spent asleep. Some people can feel exhausted even after nine hours of sleep because they have slept poorly.

Myth 4: It is possible to make up for lost sleep during the week by sleeping in during the weekends.

The Facts: This can help but only to a minimum. It cannot completely make up for the sleep deprivation experienced throughout the week. It can disrupt the sleeping and waking cycles which makes it more difficult to fall asleep on time on

Saturday nights and more difficult to wake up early on Monday mornings.

Myth 5: More sleep is always healthier.

The Facts: Oversleeping can be just as harmful as sleep deprivation. Too much of anything can be potentially dangerous to a person's health. The key to staying in the best shape is moderation.

Myth 6: In cases where a person wakes up in the middle of the night and is having trouble falling back to sleep, the best course to take is to get out of bed and do something.

The Facts: Experts recommend that when a person is having trouble getting back to sleep, getting out of bed and doing something relaxing for fifteen to twenty minutes is beneficial.

Myth 7: Everyone should get eight hours of sleep every night.

The Facts: There is no specific magic number for the hours of sleep that a person needs every day. This largely depends on each person's individual needs. Some are able to get by with five hours of good sleep while others go by nine.

Myth 8: A person needs less sleep as he or she gets older.

The Facts: The amount of sleep a person needs stays more or less constant throughout one's adult life. The difference comes in the quality of sleep that one gets. Some people may experience deeper sleep as they age or some might find that they have fragmented sleep as time goes by.

Myth 9: A person is able to train his or her body to function normally with less sleep.

The Facts: The body needs a set time to recover. Lessening this recovery time will only impact the body negatively and make performance of any function poorer.

Myth 10: The brain is at rest during sleep

The Facts: The mind is still actively working to keep all the body functions in order. The body rests while the mind is still performing its basic duties.

Myth 11: Counting sheep can help you get to sleep.

The Facts: The act of counting per se does not help a person get to sleep. It is the repetitive action that helps to relax the body and bring it to a meditative state. Depending on a person's preference, any kind of relaxing imagery can help a person relax and sleep better.

Sleep Solution Tip: Truthful knowledge can do wonders. Get informed and read on the best way or ways to improve sleep and avoid sleep deprivation.

Chapter 9: Follow A Sleep-Friendly Diet

The food we eat is our body's source of fuel. Eat high quality foods and you will perform well. Choose low quality foods, however, and your body will break down like a beaten up car without gas. Unsurprisingly, food also affects our quality of sleep.

Take, for instance, the results of a 2012 study you can find in The Journal of Clinical Endocrinology and Metabolism. These revealed that those who consume food and beverages that are specifically meant to give a temporary power boost are also those who progressively gain more weight and lose more sleep.

So, let go of that afternoon cup of coffee and slice of sugary cake. Instead, follow a healthy, balanced diet that will increase your energy, whittle down your waistline, and guarantee you a good night's rest.

Here are the dietary tips to follow:

Follow a strict eating schedule.

It is important to eat meals during fixed times throughout the day, because this trains your brain to follow a system. In turn, this will also signal you to go to sleep and wake up at the same time each day.

It is easy to set schedules for meals. For instance, if you wake up at 7 a.m. each morning, aim to have breakfast at 7:30. After three hours, have a light morning snack. At around 12:30 p.m., have lunch then enjoy an afternoon snack after 3 hours. You can then have dinner at around

6:30 p.m. Finally, have a light snack or warm beverage at 9:30 p.m.

Try setting alarms to remind you first so that you can build the habits. Eventually, you will follow them more naturally.

Reduce caffeine intake.

You might argue that you need coffeeto function properly each day, but the truth is you don't, especially if you follow a healthy diet. If you really want to drink coffee, make sure to drink it only within the window that is between 9 and 10 a.m. so that it will not negatively affect your sleep later on.

Also, limit yourself to three 8-ounce cups of caffeine, according to the National Sleep Foundation.

Cut out the sugar.

Sugar is just bad for your health. It does not have any nutritional value whatsoever and all it does is temporarily spike up your blood sugar levels. While this may cause you to feel a surge of energy, it leads to a crash that will only trigger you to want even more sugar. This addiction will lead to drastically fluctuating energy levels that will keep you from getting your much needed sleep. What is worse, you will risk developing type 2 diabetes.

Instead, snack on healthier options. If you must have something sweet, choose a more natural source of sugar such as honey or maple syrup.

Eat healthy foods that promote sleep

Complex carbs are your best friend when it comes to getting you to sleep. These are in the form of whole wheat or gluten-free grains. It is also recommended to add a smidge of lean protein to help promote sleep even further. So go ahead and get a serving of brown rice, whole wheat bread, quinoa, or buckwheat noodles for dinner.

Aside from complex carbs, you should also enjoy the following foods throughout the day as they are known to contain specific natural components that help promote better sleep:

Lettuce –contains lactucarium

Kale–rich in calcium

Halibut and tuna–rich in vitamin B6

Shrimp and lobster–rich in tryptophan

Dairy products–high in calcium

Pistachio nuts –rich in vitamin B6

Walnuts –contains tryptophan

Almonds—high in magnesium

Chickpeas—high in tryptophan

Garlic —rich in vitamin B6

Herbal teas for better sleep

Since the discovery of hot herbal tea, people have been turning to it to get better quality sleep. Among the different choices out there, here is a list of the herbs that are most popular for sleep:

Chamomile

Valerian

Lavender

Peppermint

Lemon Grass

Lemon Balm

St John's Wort

Chapter 10: Throat Exercises

Throat exercises can strengthen your airway muscles, which avoid them from collapsing and blocking your airway. This consequently reduces the severity of sleep apnea and stops snoring. Try a combination of the following exercises and see results in just a short period of time.

Say each vowel (a-e-i-o-u) aloud for three minutes, repeat a few times a day.

Close your mouth and make a pursed lip (as if making a kiss). Hold for 30 seconds. Repeat several times daily.

Press your tongue against the floor of your mouth and use a toothbrush to brush top and sides. Repeat this brushing movement five times, and repeat the sequence three times a day.

Press your tongue to the roof of your mouth. Hold the position for three minutes a day.

Place a finger in your mouth and hold it against one side of your cheek. Pull in the cheek muscle. After doing this, take a rest, and do the same on the other side until you make 10 repeats. Do this sequence three times daily.

Open your mouth and move your jaw to the right. Hold this position for 30 seconds and repeat on the left side.

Purse your lips and hold them together tightly. Move your lips up then to the right, and up then to the left. Do this 10 times and repeat the sequence three times a day.

Place a balloon on your lips. Inhale through your nose. Inflate the balloon completely through your mouth.Without removing the balloon, repeat the process five times.

Place your tongue's tip behind your top front teeth. For three minutes, slide your tongue back and forth.

Open your mouth and contract your throat muscles repeatedly for 30 seconds. When looking at the mirror, you should see your uvula ("the hanging ball") moving up and down.

Doing these exercises daily is entirely hassle-free because you can incorporate them into your daily activities, such as taking a shower, working out, commuting to work, and many others. All it takes is a conscious effort to perform them with your goals in mind. Additionally, over-all physical exercises such as running, swimming, biking, doing yoga, et cetera, will not only make you physically fit and healthy but can also help treat sleep apnea or snoring. These activities tone and strengthen your muscles including those that line your throat.

Aside from those mentioned above, there are alternative remedies you can try. One method is singing. This improves the muscle tone of your throat and soft palate, preventing them from collapsing and obstructing the airway. Studies show that learning to play the didgeridoo (a native wind instrument from Australia) can give the same benefits as singing.

Chapter 11: Proven Training To Have A Healthy Sleep

Whenever there is a change that needs to be made that will effect our health then it is smart to think about the activities involved as if you are an athlete preparing for a competition. The human body is a wonderful creation because it can be improved and allowed to work better if steps are taken to allow it to function at its highest   capacity.
One of the first things to look at is the light and temperature in the room as you try to get to sleep. Night lights are a notorious cause of sleeping problems and should be eliminated or a person should institute the use of a blindfold as they prepare for sleep each night.It is very difficult to sleep when there is too much light present in the room. Dark Sturdy curtains are available to

help keep the room just the right visibility to allow a comfortable and undisturbed sleep. This type of training is simple to do and it takes common sense to implement.

The second part of the equation for a good sleeping environment is the temperature in the room. A room should be cooler rather than hotter. It is much easier to control the temperature by adding blankets than it is to take them away.In hot temperatures it can be nearly impossible to achieve any kind of sleep because a person is so uncomfortable. Chilling out in a dark room is the best environment for sleep and most often these two symptoms we can control, but some we simply can't.

Noise is another factor in the soundness of the sleep that we experience. Unwanted, loud noises that are out of the ordinary are some of the most common complained about problems that bother sleepers.Doors slamming, machines running or a person yelling can keep a person from finding the restful sleep that they need.If a person lives in an urban area then the sounds of the city can be disturbing as well.

To combat the noise factor there are several tactics that can be taken. One is to employ some sort of white noise maker that will cover up any sudden and unwanted noises of the night. Another great ploy is to use relaxing sounds from a CD or Ipodof ocean waves or a river running to both calm and relax you and cover up the unwanted sounds of the night. Many people use the time they spend falling asleep to put on a recorded book that can be a story or perhaps a self help book. Many people believe that the subconscious mind can believe all that it hears even when we are asleep.

By controlling all of these environmental issues then people can take control and attempt to improve the quality and quantity of the sleep that they get. This is a great place to start but there are also many other sleep training methods out there to improve the sleeping experience that each person faces.

Chapter 12: 7 Steps To Break The Insomnia Cycle Forever

These 7 steps to break the insomnia cycle forever will change your life.It is important to give each step the time and focus it deserves so you can get the most from it.

These steps are not a quick fix; they require some work on your part.Once you begin, stick with it, breaking the cycle of insomnia requires life style changes and dedication.

Each step is designed to change the way you think about sleep and sleeping.Behavior modification is the best way to make changes that will stick and become part of your daily routine.As you progress through the steps you will begin to realize how life changing this process is.

As your behavior changes and these steps become part of you daily routine, insomnia will become something you can change, rather than something you struggle with or cope with.

Insomnia is more common in women than it is in men.Everyone responds to circadian rhythm.The circadian rhythm is what determines your wake and sleep cycle, it is attuned to the light/dark cycles in nature.When your circadian rhythm is out of sync, you will experience insomnia.

Insomnia can be short term or long term, both will respond to behavior modification and the steps in this chapter.Remember, these steps are meant to help you change your behavior and thoughts about sleeping.Changing how you think about sleep, think about where you sleep, and the routine you follow as the day winds down will make an impact on your life, and break the insomnia cycle.

Step 1

Regular Sleep and Wake Up Times

I know what you are thinking,"how can I establish regular sleep and wake up times if I am experiencing insomnia!", well there is an answer for that.

Snapping your fingers and announcing when you will go to bed and when you wake up is not going to establish anything; changing how you think about sleep can.

Interestingly enough, our thoughts can actually change the way we think and behave.Setting a time to go to bed and a time to wake up will help reset your circadian rhythm and help you on your way to meet the sandman.

Establish a time to go to bed that will give you at least 8 hours of sleep before you have to wake up for work.

The time you set is symbolic as well as a command for your subconscious to focus on.Once you have a sleep time that you are happy with, decide on a wake up time.

As you decide on a wake up time, think about how much time you woul

d like to have before you have to leave for work.Give yourself enough time to wake up and start your day without rushing or starting off stressed.

Your sleep and wake times must be thought of as an essential part of your daily routine, these times are as important to your wellbeing as the meals you eat and the job you perform at work or school.You must put positive thought behind these times that you have chosen, and you must tell yourself just how important they are.

These positive thoughts about sleeping and waking will eventually take hold in your subconscious and help you in your battle against insomnia.

Think about it, you probably already have a round about time to go to sleep and it probably stresses you because you know you are not going to be sleepy or you have brought your work home with you and you are stressing about completing it before you turn in.

You probably also have a slew of negative thoughts and emotions about waking up.You stress about not hearing the alarm clock, not getting enough sleep before the alarm goes off...the list is endless.

All of these negative thoughts about going to sleep and waking up make an impact on your subconscious and eventually on your circadian rhythm.

Now, choose two good times, times that provide you with a full 8 hours of sleep and time to wake up and start your day stress free, no rushing!

Do not stress about anything that involves your sleep time or your wake time; this may be tough at first, but things will fall into place.

The next step is going to help you stick to your established sleep and wake times without causing you any anxiety or stress.

Step 2

Prepare for Sleeping

This is a very important step, preparing for sleep will become a routine, and routines are behaviors that help you get things done the way you want them done.

Routine is repetition, repetition becomes habit, and habit paves the way for behavioral modification that will either benefit you and your agenda or not.

The point is, you are going to be in control of your behavior and the results; no more wishing or complaining, it's time to be doing.

Preparing for sleep involves creating a routine that helps you relax, grow sleepy, and go to bed ready to fall off to sleep.Your routine will involve positive thoughts, emotions, and associations that will put you in the mood to fall asleep.

This preparation routine will change how you think about going to sleep, and how you feel when you climb into bed.

Make a list of things you like to do that help you relax.Maybe reading a book, a relaxing scented bath, some meditation, or a hobby you enjoy.As you create the list, write down how you feel when you think about these relaxing things.

Write down your thoughts and emotions next to the things that help you relax.Now set aside at least an hour for engaging in one of these things each night before you turn in.

This hour you have set aside is probably the most important change you are going to make.When the time arrives to relax and enjoy personal time before bed don't let anything get in the way.

Read what you wrote about how this activity relaxes you and gives you a peaceful moment during your day.Don't leave out the part about reading what you wrote, it is important to reinforce the positive thoughts and emotions associated with this activity.The next step will support this step and help you stick to the routine.

Step 3

Make Your Bedroom a Sleeping Paradise

Where you sleep can really change your sleep life.Take time and create a space that is dedicated to sleep and sleep only (and sex of course).No TV in the bedroom, this may be a difficult thing to come to terms with but there can be no TV watching in sleep paradise.

This list will help you create your ultimate sleeping paradise:

No television in the room

No computer in the room

Decorate with calming colors, nothing distracting or stimulating

Pay attention to textures, colors, and patterns in your bedroom

Keep the room cool, it is easier to sleep in cool temperatures

It is important not to watch television or work/play on the computer in the bedroom.Keep the room dark when you sleep, light can affect the natural circadian rhythm.If you room gets light from neighbors, street lights, or road lights, try room darkening shades/curtains to keep the light from disturbing you.

Artificial light, especially blue light, they type of light that comes from televisions and computers disrupts melatonin production.Melatonin is a hormone involved in regulating sleep.Amber tinted glasses have been proven to reduce the amount of blue light to your eyes; wearing these glasses at night before bed can reduce the amount of blue light and keep it from suppressing melatonin production.

Keeping the room cool can actually help you fall asleep.When the body begins to get ready for sleep, it begins to release heat from the core to the skin and into the environment.If the room is too warm, this process is slower to work and this can contribute to insomnia.

Step 4

Exercise and Natural Light

Add an exercise routine to your daily routine. If you already have an exercise plan or are just starting one now, make sure some of the exercise takes place outdoors.

Natural sunlight during the day will help regulate your circadian rhythm.Exercise itself is known to contribute to sleepiness at night; the more exercise and light you enjoy during the day, the better chance you will have at getting a goodnight sleep.

Your circadian rhythm is a delicate cycle, getting proper amounts of sunlight, and darkness will help regulate your inner clock and this will help you fall asleep and stay asleep.

One of the best ways to reset your circadian rhythm is to go camping.Camping and exposure to natural light and dark schedules will reset your inner clock and get you back to sleeping every night.

Step 5

Diet Changes

There is no need to change everything about your diet to help relieve insomnia.Adding some carbs to your dinner will naturally help you fall asleep.Carbs release tryptophan and this induces sleep.

If you are on a low carb diet, your diet could be contributing to your insomnia.

It is no good to eat large amounts of food before bed or drink excessively before bed.Eat at least 4 hours before bed, this gives the body time to digest before you turn in.

Adding some carbs to your last meal will release tryptophan slowly into your system and by the time you are ready for bed, you will feel naturally sleepy.

Do not eat carb laden food right before bed, eat it during your last meal to give the carbs a chance to break down and help you fall asleep.

Alcohol is a remedy everyone talks about but it is not a remedy, it is actually the enemy.Drinking alcohol before bed may get you to sleep faster than normal but it will also wake you up.

Alcohol will stimulate you and wake you up several time during the night, and this is no way to get a refreshing sleep.Eliminate alcohol and add a few carbs; this will help you sleep and stay asleep

Step 6

No More Stimulants

Remove all stimulants from your diet, this may be tough, but it will improve your sleep.No more coffee or drink decaf coffee; coffee, no matter what time of day you drink it, can have adverse effects on your sleep.Caffeine lingers in the system and can really wreak havoc with sleep.

Caffeine is in more than coffee, it is found in cola drinks, and other soft drinks so read the labels, it is in tea of all types, unless it is decaffeinated, and stay away from chocolate, chocolate has caffeine in it too.

Removing stimulants from your diet will help you regain a natural sleep wake cycle.This won't happen overnight, but it will happen.Continue using the other steps while removing stimulants from your diet and natural sleep cycles will return.

Replace those caffeine drinks with water; water is important for keeping body systems regulated, dehydration can creep up on you and it causes leg cramping, another sleep killer.

Step 7

If You Do Not Fall Asleep Get Up

If you follow all of these steps you will begin to notice a natural sleep cycle returning.While you are practicing these steps, this step will be an important one.

If you do not fall asleep within a half an hour get up.This may seem counter intuitive for someone with insomnia, but believe it or not, it will help.

Get up if you cannot sleep and leave the bedroom.Remaining in bed and trying to force yourself to sleep will only cause frustration and stimulate your thoughts; it is better to get up.

Try going to another room and reading from a book, not a digital book, a regular book; a digital book emits blue light and this light is stimulating.Try and relax and read a book or magazine, anything that is calming, nothing that will wake you up.

Once you feel tired again, go back to the bedroom and try to go to sleep again.

If All Else Fails

The steps in this book will return your natural circadian rhythm and you will once again enjoy a good night's sleep.If these steps do not work as they should, there is another alternative, seek cognitive therapy.

Cognitive therapy will address the reasons you cannot fall asleep.Sometimes there are reasons you cannot relax, and if stress is keeping you awake regardless of your best efforts, a cognitive therapist can make a difference for you.

Cognitive therapy is about learning behavioral techniques that will help you conquer your insomnia.The steps in this book are very similar to behavioral techniques but working with a cognitive therapist is one step better.Insomnia is something you can defeat, and if you need a little extra help relaxing, a cognitive therapist will help.

Another big factor for those with insomnia is health.Remember health problems can trigger insomnia; and some medications can also trigger insomnia.As discussed elsewhere in this book, be sure you don't have any underlying health problems that could be causing your insomnia.

Chapter 13: In The Room, On The Bed

Unless you like to sleep on the sofa, the floor or you are camping, the magic happens in the room and on the bed. The ambiance in the room is very important as it can be conducive to help you fall asleep faster and have a restful night, or keep you awake. Think about how you feel when you enter a messy room, and how different it is when you enter a room that is neatly organized, smells good, is quite and well lit. The same principal can be applied to the bed. Some of the best nights of sleep I had were in hotel rooms. The feeling of being surrounded by fresh clean bed sheets, fluffy pillows and mint chocolate. Anyway, you don't need to rent hotel suites all the time or have a staff on hand to keep your room clean and fresh;

here are some quick tips on how to perfect your room and bed to help you sleep faster.

Turn off the lights; try to sleep without any light in the room, or with a very dim light. Even small amounts of light interfere with your eyes and stimulate your brain when you sleep. Avoid any kind of noises. I am not referring to music or white noise. I mean noise from the street or anything in the room. Wear earplugs to cancel the noise and a facemask to cancel the light, whenever and wherever you can't control these things.

Something that I discovered that really helps me is to light up an incense candle. There are a few scents that help me, though others bother my sense of smell. Find one that you are comfortable with; match your emotions for the day with the scent. For example, I like to have lime basil and mandarin in the bathroom as the citrus smell gives me a sense of cleanliness, while in the bedroom I like to light up scented candles of magnolia and saffron. Buy a safe candleholder and fall asleep with the light of the candle flickering on the bedroom walls.

Turn off the TV, computers, cell phone and any other electronics. If possible, make your room a sacred sanctuary without any electronic gadgets - go old school. Have some books near you to read if you really can't fall asleep or like to read in bed. Turn on some nice and relaxing music to help you fall asleep. Or even nature sounds like water or forests sounds. You should play them on something that has a timer to turn off automatically.

Several recent studies have all come to the same conclusion that it is not good to handle electronic gadgets while in bed and right before you sleep. Not only it is dangerous because some may heat up and cause fires, some also emit radiation that can be harmful during prolonged periods of exposure. The light from their screen can also effect our eyes, while the excitement sparked on the brain is hard to slow down and makes it difficult to fall asleep.

Try to sleep as comfortable as you can. Find your best sleeping position and body posture. The best way to sleep is to keep your neck straight.Do not use a very high or low pillow while your body rests on the side or back. I personally like to add an extra pillow between my legs because it allows my hips to align with my body and helps to relax my back. Even though during the night I will kick the pillow to the side of the bed, it really helps me to fall asleep faster.

I personally like to sleep naked sometimes, especially during hot summer nights. Though some people can't fall sleep without their pajamas, some of us feel we have more freedom when we sleep naked. If you sleep with someone else and if they are comfortable with the proposal, sleep naked by each other. The skin contact is soothing and relaxing for many, while that warm human touch allows you to feel safe, sexy and sleepy.

Find the most comfortable way to sleep and buy comfortable nightwear that is not too tight or loose. Tight clothes can cause your body to feel trapped and prevent your blood from flowing naturally to your arms and legs. Loose sleepwear may get tangled with the bed sheets, knot itself and even make your sleeping partner uncomfortable.

Keep in mind the temperature of the room. Research suggests that the best temperature to help you fall asleep is around 65 degrees Fahrenheit, or around 18 degrees Celsius. If your room has an air conditioner or you use a heater, control its settings to keep a steady room temperature. Sleepwear is also an important factor, I usually use silk during the summer and cotton during the winter.

Buy quality bed sheets and a comfortable mattress. You spend 8 hours a day in bed or a third of your day, so why not to make a real good investment in your bed? There is a lot to choose from and a large price range. Narrow your choices considering: weight performance, additional features, price for your budget and attributes that really matter to you. A good mattress will have a good balance between firmness and bounciness. It needs to be firm to give your body a good support and they also tend to last longer. A very stiff mattress may cause damage to the skin and sore shoulders and hips, while a mattress that is not firm enough can cause back pain. Don't worry about paying out a bit more for a mattress that has an increased life span and good back support. You are worth it!

Consider the types of cloths that you purchase for sleepwear and bed sheets. Purchase materials that are more comfortable for you and to which you will not have an allergic reaction. Chose materials that do not accumulate dust easily and are easy to wash. Wash your bed sheets and pajamas frequently; it will give you such a boost of energy and confidence just by seeing a freshly prepared bed before going to sleep. And add some mint chocolates on top of the pillows, just for an extra flair of self-indulgence.

Chapter 14: Don't Stress Over Insomnia

A standout amongst the most disappointing things that we can experience is not having the capacity to rest appropriately around evening time. On the off chance that you are finding that you are hurling and turning amid the night and on the off chance that you can't keep your psyche off of unpleasant circumstances, it cannot just influence your hours amid the evening, it can influence the whole day. Despite the fact that there are a variety of things that can cause sleep deprivation, one of the more typical reasons why we encounter it is a direct result of distressing circumstances we are experiencing.

There are truly two unique sorts of dozing issues that individuals with stretch have a tendency to experience. For a few, they can't nod off when they set down and they may wind up hurling and turning, their psyches harping on things that keep them alert. There are likewise other people who tend to nod off rapidly yet that rest is soon hindered and once they are alert, they can't fall back sleeping once more. On the off chance that anxiety is denying you of the rest that you require, there are a couple of things that you might have the capacity to do to help cure it.

Extraordinary compared to other things that you can do in this circumstance is to set up your psyche to set the distressing circumstances aside for later. For no less than one hour before you go to bed, abstain from anything that would help you to remember the unpleasant issues that you are experiencing. Work on ruminating over things that are upbuilding and do some profound breathing activities to help quiet your psyche also. Amid circumstances such as these, things like hot showers, fragrance based treatment and delicate music likewise help to quiet an exhausted personality.

You ought to likewise ensure that your body is not lacking anything that it needs. In the event that you are managing alarm assaults and these are denying you of rest, you may be short on a few vitamins. Supplement with a decent multivitamin and ensure that you are getting enough B vitamins amid the day. Despite the fact that this may not absolutely take your anxiety away in light of the fact that it doesn't change nature around you, on the off chance that you find that you are freezing about nothing then this may simply be the guilty party.

Quieting your psyche and getting the rest that you require in case you're managing excessively stress can surely be a troublesome thing to do. With a tad bit of tolerance, in any case, you can increase some control over your musings and enable yourself to get the rest that you require.

WHAT CAN BREATHING DO FOR YOUR SLEEP?

One reason that we are alive is on the grounds that we relax. A great many people tend to disregard relaxing for some reason, for the most part since it is something that we manage without truly contemplating it. In the event that we are enduring somehow or another in our life, in any case, we may be astounded to discover that breathing can really help us in various ways. Not that straightforward consistently in and out breathing that we do by intuition however moderate and consider breathing that gives our body a portion of the things that we require.

Something that profound breathing activity can convey to us is assist in the event that we are managing resting scatters. In spite of the fact that it might just be one bit of the bewilder that we require with a specific end goal to conquer these issues, it absolutely is one that we should rehearse all the time. Profound breathing quiets the brain and conveys oxygen to parts of the body that might be denied of it. It likewise places us in a more casual state which can positively go far in helping us to rest better.

Sadly, the greater part of us inhale inaccurately in light of the fact that we are breathing shallow as opposed to breathing profoundly. At whatever point you are very still and breathing typically, take a gander at your stomach. On the off chance that it is going in and out, this is demonstrating to you that your stomach is working and you are breathing profoundly. On the off chance that you tend to take your breath in shallow blasts, you are not so much giving your body the oxygen that it needs.

Profound breathing activities ought to be a piece of your night custom in the event that you have a sleeping disorder. Go into a calm piece of your home and invest a tad bit of energy profoundly breathing through your nose and gradually breathing out through your mouth. Endeavor to focus on each breath that you take and drive each upsetting thoroughly considered of your brain. It might require a tad bit of investment for you to get used to doing this yet in the end, you will find that you can place yourself into a casual state.

Keep breathing profoundly yet don't over overstate it as this may really invigorate your brain to activity. Enable your brain to concentrate on positive considerations and peaceful pictures while you are relaxing. In addition to the fact that this will help you to nod off quicker, you may find that you wake up less as often as possible too.

USING YOUR BODY CHEMISTRY TO FALL ASLEEP

You may be astounded to figure out how often our body science is the guilty party at whatever point we are having a troublesome time dozing. It is not generally an excessive number of chemicals in our body but rather it might be the absence of something that we require. In the event that you are managing a sleeping disorder or having a troublesome sludge dozing in any capacity, there are a few things that you should attempt keeping in mind the end goal to develop these transported in hormones within you before you endeavor to rest. You may find that it not just encourages you to rest quicker, it might keep you sleeping for more.

The first of these chemicals that we will discuss is the hormone that is known as serotonin. Serotonin is available in our body for various distinctive reasons yet one of the fundamental things that it does is to influence us to rest easy. On the off chance that we are having a troublesome time resting in light of the fact that we tend to worry over various things previously we go to bed, serotonin may influence the adjust toward us. This hormone is discharged from our body at whatever point we practice so it is a smart thought for us to move around a tiny bit during that time keeping in mind the end goal to have a wealth of it. Trust it or not, warm drain may likewise trigger the generation of serotonin in light of the tryptophan that it contains.

Another hormone that we may require which can absolutely help us to nod off is melatonin. This is a characteristic rest hormone however a few of us might be insufficient in it for some reason. This specific hormone is accessible as a characteristic supplement and has been appeared much of the time to help people who are managing sleep deprivation. Incidentally, it likewise helps a man who has stream slack for a similar reason. It reset our organic clock and encourages us to experience the regular cycle of rest.

One last thing that you ought to do is to ensure that you have every one of the vitamins and minerals that your body needs. Taking a quality multivitamin regular might have the capacity to help you to bring your body into the adjust that it needs. You ought to likewise ensure that you are eating a lot of crude products of the soil as this will likewise go far in curing your sleep deprivation.

Chapter 15: Medications; Non Pharmacological And Pharmacological

In medicine, sleep deprivation or insomnia is broadly measured utilizing the Athens insomnia scale. It is measured utilizing eight separate parameters identified with slumber, at last it is spoken to as a general scale which evaluate a singular's sleep design A qualified slumber specialist ought to be counseled in the analysis of any slumber issue so the suitable measures can be taken. Past medicinal history and a physical examination need to be carried out to wipe out different conditions that could be the reason for the sleep deprivation. After all different conditions are precluded, a thorough slumber history ought to be taken. The slumber history ought to include slumber propensities, drugs (non-prescribed and prescribed medications), consumption of alcohol, nicotine and intake of caffeine, illnesses that are comorbid, and slumber environment. A sleep journal can be utilized to stay informed regarding the subject's sleeping patterns. The journal ought to have bed time, aggregate sleep time, time to rest onset, number of arousals, utilization of meds, and wakening time and subjective sentiments in the morning.

People who grumble of a sleeping disorder ought not to have routinely polysomnography to screen for slumber disorders. This test may be shown for patients with manifestations along with sleep deprivation, including sleep apnea, a hazardous neck width, obesity or dangerous fullness of the tissue in the oropharynx. Usually, the test is not expected to make a diagnosis, and a sleeping disorder, particularly for working individuals, can frequently be dealt with by changing work calendar, to set aside a few minutes for sufficient slumber and by enhancing slumber hygiene.

A few patients may need to do a slumber study to figure out whether sleep deprivation is present. The sleep study will include the evaluation tools of a polysomnogram and the different latent sleep tests will be directed in a precise environment. Sleep specialists are qualified to diagnose various slumber issues. Patients with different illnesses or diseases, such as delayed sleep phase syndrome, are frequently misdiagnosed with essential sleep deprivation. When an individual experiences difficulty in getting some sleep, nonetheless has a typical sleeping pattern once slept, a postponed circadian rhythm is the presumable reason.

Much of the time, insomnia is co-bleak with an alternate illness, reactions from drugs, or a mental issue. Nearly 50% of all diagnosed sleep deprivation or insomnia is identified with psychiatric disorders. Information of causation is redundant for a diagnosis.

Treatment

It is essential to recognize or discount therapeutic and mental causes before settling on the treatment for insomnia. Cognitive behavioral treatment (CBT) has been discovered to be as successful as physician recommended medicines are for transient treatment of chronic insomnia. In addition, there are evidences that the advantageous impacts of CBT, rather than those created by drugs, may last well, past the end of active treatment. Pharmacological medications have been used to lessen acute insomniac symptoms;

their part in the administration of chronic insomnia remains unclear. Several diverse sorts of solutions are additionally successful for treating sleep deprivation. In any case, numerous specialists do not prescribe sleeping pills to be used for a longer period of time. It is likewise imperative to distinguish and treat other restorative conditions that may be helping insomnia, for example, depression, breathing issues, and chronic pain

Non-pharmacological

Non-pharmacological systems have equivalent adequacy to hypnotic drug for insomnia and they may have longer enduring impacts. Hypnotic medicine is prescribed for shorter term, since the reliance with bounce back, withdrawal impacts upon suspension or resistance can develop.

Non pharmacological systems give reliable improvements to sleep deprivation and are suggested as a first line and long haul methodology for treatment. The methods incorporate thoughtfulness regarding slumber cleanliness, boost control, behavioral intercessions, sleep restriction treatment, patient relaxation and education therapy. Reducing the temperature of blood streaming to the cerebrum moderates the mind's metabolic rate decreasing insomnia. Some illustrations are; keeping a diary, limiting the time spending alert in couch, rehearsing relaxation practices, and keeping up a consistent slumber calendar and a wake-up time. Behavioral treatment can support a patient in creating new rest practices to enhance rest quality and consolidation. Behavioral treatment may incorporate, learning sound slumber propensities to advance slumber relaxation, experiencing light treatment to help with stress-lessening methods and managing the circadian clock.

EEG biofeedback has exhibited viability in the treatment of sleep deprivation with upgrades in length of time and nature of sleep.

Sleep hygiene is a typical term for the majority of the practices which can be related to improved slumber. These practices are utilized as the premise of slumber intercessions and are the essential center of sleep instruction programs. Behaviors incorporate the utilization of stimulant, nicotine and liquor utilization, expanding the consistency and proficiency of slumber scenes, minimizing medication use and daytime resting, the increase in normal activity, and the help of a positive slumber environment. Exercise can be useful in maintaining sleep routine however ought not to be carried out near to the time of rest. The making of a positive slumber environment might likewise be useful in diminishing the effects of insomnia. So as to create a positive slumber environment, one ought to remove stuff that can result in stress or distressful thoughts.

Prevention

Sleep deprivation can be transient or long haul. Aversion of the slumber issue may involve updating a steady sleeping calendar, for example, waking up and resting at the same times consistently. Additionally, one ought to keep away from beverages with caffeine amid the 8 hours prior to resting time. While activity is vital and can help the sleeping process, it is critical to not practice just before time to bed, in this way making a smoothing environment. In conclusion, one's bed ought to be for slumber and sex. These are a portions of slumber hygiene to be focused on. Going to rest and awakening the same time consistently can make a relentless example, which may help against insomnia.

Medications

Numerous light sleepers depend on dozing tablets and different tranquilizers to get rest. In a few spots prescriptions are endorsed to in excess of 95% of restless person cases. The rate of grown-ups utilizing a medicine tranquilizer increments with age. Amid 2005–2010, around 4% of U.S. grown-ups, 20 years and over, reported that they took medicine tranquilizers in the previous 30 days. Intake was decreased with the decreasing age (those matured 20–39) at around 2%, increased to 6% among those with 50–59 years of age, and arrived at 7% among those of 80 years and over. More grown-up ladies (5.0%) reported utilizing medicine tranquilizers than elderly men (3.1%). Non-Hispanic white grown-ups reported higher utilization of tranquilizers (4.7%) than non-Hispanic dark (2.5%) and Mexican-American (2.0%) adults. No distinction was demonstrated between non-Hispanic dark elders and Mexican-American grown-ups. As an option to taking physician recommended medications, some confirmation demonstrates that a normal individual looking for transient help may discover alleviation from assuming control over-the-counter antihistamines, for example, diphenhydramine or doxylamine. Certain classes of tranquilizers, for example, benzodiazepines and more updated non-benzodiazepine medications can likewise cause physical reliance, which shows in withdrawal side effects if the medication is not deliberately lowered. The benzodiazepine and non-benzodiazepine hypnotic drugs likewise have various reactions, for example, day time weakness, engine vehicle crashes, cognitive impairments and falls and breaks. Elderly individuals are touchier to these side-effects. The non-benzodiazepines zolpidem and zaleplon have not showed enough viability in slumber upkeep. A few benzodiazepines have showed viability in slumber upkeep in the fleeting yet in the more drawn out term are connected with resistance and reliance. Sedates that may demonstrate more successful and more secure than existing medications for sleep deprivation is a zone of dynamic research.

Alternative Medicines

A few light sleepers use herbs, for example, Withania somnifera, lavender, bounces cannabis, valerian, chamomile, and passion flower. L-Arginine L-aspartate, S-adenosyl-L-homocysteine, and delta slumber inciting peptide (DSIP) may be additionally useful in reducing insomnia. A recent report distributed in Psychopharmacologia found that orally controlled THC altogether diminished slumber idleness and recurrence of slumber intrusions in 9 solid subjects. A 20 mg dosage of THC was discovered to be best, decreasing slumber idleness by over an hour on average. A recent report distributed in Anesthesia and Analgesia found that engineered THC was more successful than the stimulant amitriptyline at enhancing slumber quality in patients with fibromyalgia. However, visit THC utilization has been demonstrated to cause undesirable identity changes and propensities so it ought to be stayed away from. Sanitized valerian extricate has experienced different studies and has all the earmarks of being unobtrusively effective.

Chapter 16: Symptoms Of Sleep Disorder

Sleep can serve as a barometer of your overall health. Sleep disorder can interfere with your personal and professional life. People who sleep well are said to be healthier than those who suffer sleep disorders.

Unfortunately, even a small amount of sleep loss can cause a negative effect on a person's performance. It is important for people to understand that sleep is a necessity and not a luxury. People who have been dealing with sleep disorders for a long time may already find it normal to feel sleepy during the day and have difficulty sleeping at night.

The first step in overcoming sleep disorder is by identifying the symptoms and then making changes to your sleeping habits.

Symptoms of Sleep Disorder

It is important to differentiate occasional sleep problems from the symptoms of sleep disorder. Here are some of the telltale sign of sleep deprivation.

o Irritability

o Experiences Difficulty Staying Still

o Difficulty Concentrating

o Feels Tired Everyday

o Requires Caffeine to Function Throughout the Day

o Slow Reaction

o Dry and Flaky Skin

o Emotionally Imbalanced

3 Different Sleep Disorders

There are over 70 sleep disorders and most of them can be managed successfully. Here are the most common sleep disorders and some of the treatments available.

Insomnia

Insomnia is the most common type of sleeping disorder. It is described as the inability to get enough amount of sleep. Most people with insomnia report feeling stressed after waking up.

Insomnia almost always has a deeper cause such as stress, depression or anxiety. It can also be caused by poor lifestyle like unhealthy diet and lack of exercise. Insomnia can be categorized depending on how long and often it occurs. Acute insomnia is short term and can last from one night to few weeks. Chronic insomnia is longer and can happen at least three nights a week.

Treatment

Acute or occasional insomnia may not require a specific treatment. Mild insomnia can be cured with lifestyle changes and by practicing good sleeping habits. Doctors can also prescribe a sleeping pill which you can use for a limited time.

Keep in mind that prolonged use of sleeping pill can negatively affect the body. Avoid buying over the counter sleeping pills because these may cause unwanted side effects and may lose effectiveness over time.

Chronic insomnia can be cured by treating the underlying condition that is causing the problem. A psychologist can recommend an effective therapy like behavioral therapy which can help you identify the activities that can worsen your insomnia. Relaxation exercise and sleep restriction therapy also work.

Sleep Apnea

Sleep apnea is a common sleeping disorder that happens when a person's breathing stops because of blocked air passages. The body responds by disturbing your sleep in order to start your breathing again. It is usually followed by choking and gasping sounds. Other symptoms include frequent pauses in breathing and nasal congestions.

People might not even remember waking up, but they will feel exhausted and restless during the day. Sleep apnea is a serious condition and can be life-threatening. The classifications of this condition include central, obstructive, and complex sleep apnea.

Central sleep apnea. This is a disorder where a person's breathing repeatedly stops and resumes during sleep. It happens when the central nervous system does not succeed in controlling the muscles involved in breathing.

Obstructive sleep apnea. This occurs when the airway is temporarily blocked. Because of this, a person usually wakes up with a loud gasp or body jerking. This is accompanied by loud snoring.

Complex sleep apnea. This is a condition where people develop two types of sleep apnea at the same time.

Treatment

Being diagnosed with sleep apnea can be frightening, but it is a treatable condition. Self-help treatment can help people with mild sleep apnea. Home remedies and lifestyle changes can also reduce the symptoms. Moderate and severe sleep apnea should be treated with the help of a medical professional. They can evaluate your symptoms and explore treatment options.

CPAP or Continuous Positive Airflow Pressure is the common treatment for sleep apnea. It is a device with a mask that keeps the air passage open while a person sleeps.

People who are overweight have higher tendencies of sleep apnea. The extra tissue at the back of their throat may block the airway while they sleep. Smoking is also believed to contribute in fluid retention which can increase inflammation in the throat.

Here are some exercises that can help control sleep apnea.

• Press your tongue at the floor of your mouth and brush it with a toothbrush. Repeat five times, three times a day.

• Hold a finger against your cheek and pull the cheek muscle. Repeat 10 times.

• Hold your tongue at the roof of your mouth for three minutes.

• Purse your lips and move it right and left. Repeat it three times.

Restless Legs Syndrome

Restless leg syndrome is characterized by the irresistible urge to move the limbs. This usually occurs when the person is lying down. Common signs include the uncomfortable sensation in the legs accompanied by the strong urge to move them. This can also be triggered by inactivity and can be worst during the night. Restless legs syndrome is hereditary and is more common among elderly people. Here are some home remedies to make the syndrome more bearable.

Treatment

Heat and Cold massage. One of the easiest home remedy for restless leg syndrome is the application of warm and cold packs to the muscles. You can alternate the heat and cold application. You can also soak your legs in warm water and massage it. Exercise and relaxation. Performing light and moderate exercise during the day can help you sleep at night. However, be careful not to overdo it.

It is also essential to dedicate some time to stretching. Stress and muscle tension can contribute to restless leg syndrome. Try to relax your muscles through mediation and yoga. Over the counter medicine. People who experience occasional symptoms of the disorder should use over the counter medications to ease the pain.

You can use pain relievers like acetaminophen drugs. However, do not rely on these drugs because these can cause some side effects like stomach ache and ulcers.

Dietary supplements. Restless leg syndrome can be caused by vitamin deficiencies. A blood test can help you determine what vitamins and minerals you need and your doctor can prescribe the right supplement for you.

Avoid staying in a single position for too long. It is important to move your body often to avoid the symptoms of restless leg syndrome. Also, avoid drinks that contain caffeine such as coffee and soft drinks.

Narcolepsy

Narcolepsy is a sleeping disorder that causes uncontrollable daytime drowsiness. It is caused by a dysfunction in the brain that controls the sleep and waking. People with narcolepsy may suddenly sleep while talking or standing. People can also start dreaming even before they are fully asleep. Narcolepsy also causes people to lose control of their muscles whenever they are experiencing strong emotions.

Treatment

There has still been no cure for narcolepsy, but a combination of self-help treatment and counseling can enable patients to enjoy normal daily activities.

Counseling and support group. Most people with narcolepsy are also exhibiting signs of depression. Most patients would be embarrassed because of their lack of body control. You can reach out to psychologists and treatment centers to reduce the sense of isolation that you might feel.

Take naps during the day. Schedule a 15-minute nap during the day and try to sleep at the same hour every night. This can prevent you from falling asleep unintentionally.

Avoid caffeine because this can interrupt your normal sleep pattern. Alert your family, friends and co-workers about your condition so that they may offer help when needed. Carry a tape recorder to capture any conversation in case you fall asleep and forget.

Break larger tasks into smaller ones. Focus on one thing at a time to avoid feeling overwhelmed.

Circadian Rhythm Sleep Disorder

Every person has their own biological clock that regulates their sleep and waking pattern. This can also be called as circadian rhythms. A humans' biological clock is primarily influenced by light. Once the sun is up, the brain sends a signal to the body that it is time to wake up. When there is less light, melatonin is released which triggers the brain to sleep.

Once your circadian rhythm is disturbed, you feel disoriented and sleepy. The disruption of circadian rhythm is also associated with other sleep disorder.

The most common type of circadian sleep disorder is jet lag. It happens when a person travels into another country with a different time zone.

Symptoms may include sleepiness, headache and stomach problems. The direction of the flight may also influence the symptoms. Flying east causes worst jet lag than flying west.

Treatment

It may take some time for your body to reset its internal clock. Here are some tips in preventing and coping with jet lag.

You can prevent jet lag by gradually adjusting your sleep habit three days before your flight. For the first day, sleep 30 minutes before your usual bedtime.

On the second day, sleep one hour earlier. On the third day, sleep 90 minutes earlier.

After a long trip, do not sleep until it is bedtime in the new time zone. Spend as much time outside and let your skin absorb sunlight to reset your biological clock. Drink water but avoid caffeine. Caffeine can dehydrate the body and worsen the symptoms of jet lag.

Shift Work Sleeping Problem

Shift work sleeping problem can happen if your work schedule and biological clock is not in tune with one other. Many people work during night and early morning shift. This may force the body to work when it naturally wants to sleep. Other people may adjust better to the change while some may have difficulty adapting to their new schedule. People who work during the night get less quality of sleep than those who work regular shift. This can result to sleep deprivation and lack of productivity.

Treatment

Take regular breaks and try to minimize the frequency of shift changes. If possible, request for a later schedule than earlier to make it easier for you to adjust later on. Regulate your sleep pattern by exposing yourself to bright lights at work and dimming the lights when it's time to sleep.

Delayed Sleep Phase Disorder

Delayed sleep phase disorder happens when the biological clock of a person is significantly delayed. People who experience this sleeping problem wake up and rise later than most people. Delayed sleep phase disorder makes it difficult for people to function effectively in normal hours like attending morning classes and coming to work at 9 o' clock.

Treatment

Bright light therapy. Exposing yourself to bright light for 30 minutes can help reset your body clock. Ask your doctor if there are commercially available light boxes that you can use. Avoiding light at night. Any light can theoretically delay the sleep pattern of an individual. Avoid light coming from the computer or the TV one hour before your bed time.

Chapter 17: The History And Facts About Insomnia

What Effects Does Insomnia have on our Health?

Sleep is not a new idea for us. In fact, sleep has always been needed for humans and animals in order to survive. For humans, it is a little more important. There have been references to sleep made for thousands of years. The Bible and the Babylonian Talmud both mention sleep quite frequently. Problems with sleeping are mentioned in these texts as well. In some written works, authors use words to describe their sleep patterns, which sound quite a bit like narcolepsy.

We all know that sleep disorders are not new to us, but technology has made it easier to find them and treat them. Sleep research began in the 1800's. Reports tell us that sleep scientist, Richard Caton, was one of the first to do research on small animals while they were sleeping. They eventually helped him to learn more about the stages of our sleep cycles. Just a few years after the research that Caton did, medical books first described narcolepsy. It wasn't until the 20th century that more research was being done on sleep disorders and even more became named and classified.

With insomnia being the most common sleep disorder, it is usually temporary and about 30% of people that are diagnosed with it. No one really knows exactly when it was properly discovered, but it is pretty evident that people haven't been getting the right amount of sleep and this was probably happening thousands of years ago too.

Narcolepsy was mentioned all the way back to texts dating in the 15th century. In 1937, non-REM sleep disorders were discovered. Alfred Loomis began to do more research on sleep terrors and sleepwalkers. There has been so much research done on the various sleep disorders and as you have seen, there is no known cure for many of them. As we continue to dive into these disorders, here are some of the most interesting facts about insomnia.

Facts About Insomnia

Most of us don't get enough sleep, but does that always mean that we are suffering from insomnia? Not necessarily, but if you do suffer from insomnia, it will not last very long unless there is another medical condition that goes along with it. The effects of losing sleep can be crippling. Our jobs and our relationships will suffer.

There are many facts about insomnia that may help you to figure out why you have it.

There have been a small number of insomnia cases, where the sufferer has died. This type of insomnia is called Familial Fatal Insomnia and it is very rare, but it can cause a person to never fall asleep. This can result in death. Familial Fatal insomnia causes the sleeper to never get enough sleep to keep their brain functions working correctly. This then causes the loss of mental functions and coordination. This is an inherited form of insomnia and death will come anywhere from eight to 75 months after it has been diagnosed.

The symptoms of Familial Fatal insomnia can start by having small difficulties falling asleep and staying asleep. Sometimes, the sleeper will notice spasms while they are sleeping. Their body may move a lot during sleep with kicking and punching being part of their sleep. Soon, they will begin to experience loss of coordination and mental functions will slowly start to deteriorate. The heart rate and blood pressure may increase too. So far, there have been no known treatments, but doctors can help to find ways to help the sufferer sleep as much as possible.

Insomnia is a sleep disorder that can cause more than the loss of sleep and energy. Insomnia can also cause drug and alcohol abuse. Many people who can't sleep will turn to alcohol and drugs that are depressants, to help them to find sleep. This is how many sufferers start to get dependent on these substances.

Effects of Insomnia on Health

There are millions of people who suffer from insomnia. Doctors often overlook it, but for those who deal with it nightly, it can really take a toll on the body and the mind. Most of us require about seven to eight full hours of sleep each night to function properly. If this is disrupted in any way, we will start to feel it almost instantly. Not only does the lack of sleep make us foggy, but it can also cause our emotions to escalate even further. Here are a few effects that losing sleep can have on us.

Being tired can cause accidents. Strangely enough, historians often blame sleep deprivation on a lot of disasters such as Three Mile Island, the Exxon Valdez oil spill, and the Chernobyl nuclear meltdown. How did sleepiness have anything to do with these accidents? Three Mile Island nuclear plant is in Pennsylvania. Sleep deprivation was to blame for this disaster because the workers were getting very little sleep and did not notice some small flaws in the reactor. They did not see that coolant was escaping and this caused a chain reaction in the reactor. By not seeing what was happening, because they were too focused on being exhausted, the reactor ended up overheating. Luckily, there were only small injuries from this and no deaths occurred.

The Exxon Valdez oil spill is blamed on sleep deprivation because the captain of the vessel had had very little sleep after a long night of drinking. The man steering the vessel had been awake for over 18 hours. The entire crew had been complaining of fatigue and being overworked.

Lastly, Chernobyl has been blamed for sleep deprivation. The workers at the plant were working at least 12 hours a day because they had to meet strict guidelines. When investigators were looking into this accident, they blamed it on the fatigue of the staff.

Losing sleep is very dangerous when it comes to driving as well. Being tired can slow down your reaction time and cause you to crash your car if you do fall asleep at the wheel. Workers who have to put in long hours on the job are excessively tired and tend to have more accidents at work.

Health problems can arise if you are not getting the proper amount of sleep. Heart problems, high blood pressure, strokes, and diabetes can all be caused by insomnia. Along with these conditions, insomnia can kill your sex drive. Losing sleep lowers your libido and interest in sex altogether. With very little energy, men and women both may be thinking more about sleep than sex with their partner.

Losing sleep is often associated with obesity too. The less sleep you are getting at night can be the reason that you are overweight. Losing sleep is often associated with having lowered levels of leptin. This is a hormone that helps to curb your appetite and is produced when you are sleeping. When you stop getting the right amount of sleep, the production of leptin drops. This causes you to be hungry practically all day. We all know overeating causes obesity so these two go hand in hand.

As you can tell insomnia and sleep deprivation can cause some catastrophes in our lives and in our world. Think about how Chernobyl would be a much better place to live if the meltdown wouldn't have happened and if the workers just got a little more sleep. It is pretty crazy to think that insomnia can cause these huge problems. It is possible to treat insomnia with natural methods and these methods give us hope that we won't encounter any more disasters because we will all be getting the right amount of sleep each night.

Chapter 18: Sleep Destroying Habits And How To Break Them

Sleep quality is essential. Humans spend one-third of their lives sleeping. Consider how you plug your electronic devices into the mains to recharge. Sleep s your charger and it helps you regenerate and recharge your batteries.

These are the most common reasons that our sleep patterns are disrupted:

• Stress

In our busy world stress is the number one killer of the 21st century. We are all guilty of lying in our bed worrying about work, relationships and other factors in our lives. Clearing your mind may seem impossible, but it is essential that you go to bed with a stress-free mind. Watch a humorous clip online or read a funny quote. Does a particular activity always make you smile? Make sure you do it before you go to bed. Your state of mind should be optimistic and carefree. Worrying about cash or work will not solve anything, it will only leave you tired and irritable in the morning.

● Poor mental activity

Intense light prevents the body from producing melatonin and stimulates the mind. Switch off the TV or computer screen and practice a restorative action instead. Read a book using an incandescent lamp or take a gentle walk in the garden. Practice yoga or meditation before bedtime and feel the benefit of a calm mind and a relaxed body.

● Room temperature

This is a personal choice should be tailored to the individual. People have an internal physical clock that regulates your core temperature. Your body needs to be cool when sleeping as heat tells your inner clock that it is time to get up. If your body warms up in the middle of the night you will automatically wake. There is no optimum temperature that works for everyone as we all have different metabolisms. Make sure your room is at the right temperature for you and feel the benefits while you sleep.

● Supplements and medication

We have already discussed the caffeine in some pain restrictors, but there are other drugs that can affect your sleep. Steroids and beta-blockers can contain stimulants and affect your sleep and keep you awake at night. Vitamin B supplements should be taken before 2 p.m. to avoid it disrupting your sleep. Whenever you are prescribed new medications or are considering additional supplements, ask your doctor or pharmacist to make sure your sleep will not be affected.

• Exposure to artificial light

How often have you been on your computer or smartphone just before bedtime and all you can see when you close your eyes is a screen? You need to prioritize your sleep and shun the devices. Artificial lights combined with the poor mental activity we have already mentioned are key factors to sleep deprivation.

• Eating too much food

When you have a busy schedule, it can be tempting to eat a huge meal once you get home and then go to bed. Socializing can also involve eating later than normal and going to sleep with a full stomach. Heartburn and lack of digestion will disturb your sleeping patterns and keep you awake.

Sometimes we need to sleep even when we are not tired. If you follow the tips that we have covered but are still wide awake what can you do to fall asleep?

● Play soothing music: Create a playlist with songs that have a slow rhythm (60 to 80 beats a minute) and listen for 30 minutes before falling to sleep. There is a list of suitable songs on Spotify named the 20 most streamed tracks for sleep. Avoid ear buds or headphones and invest in pillow speakers.

● Breathe only through your left nostril: Are you aware that during the day you alternate your breathing between your left and right nostril? When you breathe through your right nostril you are more alert and when you breathe through your left nostril you feel relaxed and calmer. Induce sleep and relaxation by actively breathing through your left nostril using the following techniques:

▪ Block your right nostril with your right thumb

▪ Take long, steady breaths through your left nostril

▪ Repeat and continue for up to 10 minutes until it feels like you are dominantly using your left nostril

▪ Sleep on your right side to help your left nostril breathe freely

● Dipping your face in cold water: We have already discovered that a lower body temperature helps induce sleep. If you are wide awake, try filling a sink with cold water and some cold packs from the freezer. Immerse your face for 30 seconds and this will make your blood pressure and heart rate to drop. This technique is known as Cold Thermogenesis and is a tried and tested way to sleep when not tired.

● Use Acupressure: The therapy of acupressure involves the placing of fingers with levels of pressure on specific points of the body. Normally a massage therapist would administer acupressure, but this simple method can be self-administered using the following method:

▪ Locate the acupressure point known as the Inner Gate. This is the central point of the inner side of the forearm, two and a half fingers from the crease at your wrist.

▪ Stimulate the point by placing the right thumb on the inner side of your left wrist and apply pressure for 90 seconds. Change position by applying pressure to the same point on the opposite arm for 90 seconds. Repeat until you feel relaxed.

There are many different points to use acupressure depending on the result you wish to achieve. Natural methods like acupressure and reflexology help us to achieve improved sleep without resorting to medicinal aids.

These hacks will all benefit your sleep and when combined with a healthy diet and exercise routine will enhance your overall wellbeing. If you suffer from insomnia you will feel sluggish, melancholy and can also be lacking in focus. Your health can suffer, and you risk suffering from diabetes, cancer, coronary illness, and diminished libido.

Chapter 19: Sleep Boosters

Having seen the importance of sleep and what we should avoid for a better night's sleep, let's look at some of the things we should do to improve our sleep.

Exercise

Exercise is vitally important to keep us fit and healthy. It's not surprising that exercise helps us sleep better at night. There are several reasons for this. The first one is that exercise raises our core body temperature. It takes some time for the temperature to get back to normal levels and this aids in our sleeping. The temperature gets down even lower than if we hadn't exercised, making us sleep soundly. We generally sleep better when our core body temperature is lower. We should strive to exercise about five hours before sleep or earlier. Having exerting exercises right before bed can be counterproductive. It stimulates the body and mind and according to what we have seen earlier, we don't want to do this right before we sleep. It also raises our core body temperature. We can't find sleep in this state. If you can't find time for this kind of exercise you can have some light exercise such as stretching and yoga right before bed. These will be helpful as well.

The relationship between exercise and sleep is mutually beneficial. When we exercise we sleep better and when we sleep better, we are able to exercise better. Have you ever just felt too tired to exercise, this might have been caused by a poor night's sleep. The best time to have some exercises to improve on your sleep is late afternoon and early evening. This will give your body enough time to lower the core body temperature before bedtime.

Morning exercises are also beneficial in that they improve our mood throughout the day, keep us more focused and ultimately, this helps us sleep better at night.

There are no specific exercises we can say are good for us when it comes to aiding sleep. Any exercise is good exercise. What we should ensure is that it is vigorous and raises our heart rate. Cardiovascular exercises for instance do this very well. You can run, brisk walk or swim. You don't have to go to the gym. You could also put some music on and dance vigorously in your house just make sure you can feel your heart beat faster. 20 minutes of vigorous exercise each day will work wonders for your sleep and your heath in general.

Napping

Most people need a nap during the day, if time and your schedule allows. There has always been a debate on whether a nap is beneficial to us or not. Most recently, there has been a conclusion that a nap is good for us. But we have to take it at the right time. Have you ever found yourself dozing off in a meeting or lacking concentration while doing some work? The solution is not getting a distraction or some fresh air, its time you took a short nap and got refreshed. Our body temperature has two main dips during the day. The first is around 8 hours after we wake up. This makes us feel sleepy and a nap at this time would be very productive for us. The second dip is actually when we are about to go to bed. So around 8 hours after you wake up, you can have a nap. This translates to early afternoon. However, it's not disastrous of you don't take one. What's disastrous is having a nap any other time as this will greatly affect your sleep pattern at night. The duration of the nap should be no longer than 30 minutes. Even if you don't feel sleepy, simply resting whilst closing your eyes will improve your concentration levels later in the afternoon. To emphasize the effect of a nap, take an example of kids, they usually nap during the day and even if they later engage in a boring activity, they will not doze off, they just become restless.

Diet

Diet has an effect on every bodily function. We are in essence what we eat. When we feed poorly, we suffer, and sleep will be one area where the effect will be heavily felt. A balanced diet full of vegetables and fruits will do wonders for our sleep. Include low fat protein, whole grains and adequate amounts of water in your diet. Cut down on the junk and rather, snack on fruits. When we are full of health, our body functions well and we sleep better. One of the leading causes of insomnia and other sleeping conditions is poor health. When we suffer from common infections and chronic conditions, we do not sleep well.

Our eating routine affects our quality of sleep too. Most people take a light breakfast, moderate lunch and a heavy dinner. This shouldn't be the case. For a better sleep we should aim to have a heavy meal in the morning, moderate lunch and a light dinner. This has been shown to the best mode of eating for our health and in our case for a better night's sleep. A heavy meal in the evening overloads our system as it tries to digest this food. We might feel bloated, suffer heartburn or even need to wake up in the middle of the night to visit the washroom. Adjust to the more sleep friendly routine.

Having the right mattress

If there is one item we should put a lot of thought in when making a purchase is our mattress. This is because you spend at least 8 hours each day on it. This is a lot of time. And what's more, you don't get to change a mattress each day as we do with our clothes and shoes. It's sad, that most people will have a poor quality mattress while they spend a lot of money on other not very essential items. We only get to think about the mattress when it's already very old, and has caused us many bad nights. Even when we buy the mattress, we look at the top cushioning rather than the padding.

When buying a mattress consider the type, firmness and size. In firmness, don't go for the soft and fluffy. That would be a bad choice. Go for a firm mattress that's not soft. It's should not contain depressions and bumps. In fact, when you lie, it shouldn't take the entire shape of your body. On the other hand don't go for a rock for a mattress. The best one should be gently supportive. When you have used a mattress and has developed some bumps, it's time to get a new one. The average lifespan of a mattress is 10 years. There are many types of mattresses but the recommend one is one made with innerspring. They have some steel coils, insulation and padding. They are firm and will support your body adequately. The main advantage they have over other mattresses is that they breathe well at night and thus offer a cooler environment. Our bodies lose a lot of moisture at night and when a mattress doesn't soak up this moisture and circulate it, we end up sweaty and hot. In terms of size, go for a big mattress. You don't wish to have a limited space while you sleep especially if you share the bed with a partner. We need to feel we can toss around freely as we want. You might be surprised to know that you move up to 30 times in a night. When you have a small bed, you subconsciously limit this movement and this affects your sleep.

When buying a mattress, you should take your time and be as picky as possible. Do not settle for anything. Most stores will allow you try out the mattress before you buy. Lie on it and take your time. Sleep in your preferred position for a few minutes to feel it out. Better still, ask them if they offer a try period after you buy where you can return and exchange the mattress if you don't like it

Chapter 20: Can Hypnotherapy Help?

Hypnotherapy is a procedure wherein changes are introduced into a person's thoughts and behaviors via suggestion. Also referred to as hypnosis, it is actually a trance-like state of mind wherein the patient is put in a level of deep relaxation and openness to suggestion. It is a procedure that taps into the deepest recesses of the patient's subconscious.

Hypnosis was derived from the name of the Greek God of sleep, *Hypnos*, which literally means sleep. However, hypnosis is not a form of sleep but rather a deep state of increased concentration. The procedure is a way of communicating ideas to the subconscious.

Hypnotherapy aims to change your behavioral patterns. Through suggestion and conditioning, negative thoughts and patterns are replaced with positive patterns. Most sleeping problems are brought about by stress and anxiety. In order to release these negative emotions, you have to replace them with positivity. Accessing your subconscious during your most relaxed stage helps in eliminating these negative thoughts and introducing new and positive ideas.

Hypnosis can help treat insomnia, sleep terrors, and sleepwalking.

The success of hypnotherapy depends on the following factors:

The patient's pre-hypnotic beliefs, thoughts, intentions, and expectations

The patient's ability to think and absorb suggestions

Ability of the patient to create a bond with the hypnotherapist while undergoing treatment

Ability to interpret suggestions and therapeutic methods

Techniques Used to Treat Insomnia

Hypnotherapists help patients go into the self-hypnosis state wherein they can induce a level of physical floating relaxation. If patients have uncomfortable thoughts, they can easily project these thoughts onto a different plane, like an imaginary screen, while they are in a trance-like state. Patients are able to facilitate their own thoughts, throwing away the negatives and using all the positives.

Visualization is another technique that is commonly used. Patients are asked to see themselves sitting by the river as they are made to observe as the water flows. They are instructed to place their thoughts on the leaves that are floating on the water. This process allows patients to let go of their thoughts until they are totally relaxed, body and soul.

Alternatively, patients can be asked to see themselves among the clouds observing how the winds carry them away until they achieve that level of ultimate relaxation.

Hypnotherapy Techniques for Sleep Terrors

Since sleep terrors are common among children, hypnotherapists suggest that parents stay with their children at bedtime. When a child shows signs of sleepiness, the parent can start giving positive suggestions to the child, like the parents will be there to keep the child safe. Children have to always be reminded that they will never be alone and that their parents will never leave them.

Chapter 21: Top Techniques To Boost Health And Help Your Body Sleep Better

The HCCH cure is effective since it also takes health into account. This chapter is not about general tips on health, although it is a given that health is an important factor as well – it is about specific information related to health, lifestyle,and diet that would help you get a good sleep.

Which Micronutrients Matter to You

Before stuffing your fridge with all sorts of fruits and vegetables, or investing in several dozen bottles' worth of nutritional pills, you have to know which micronutrients really have slumber-enhancing properties. Magnesium is one such substance.

While it's not completely understood how magnesium regulates sleep (most likely it has something to do with its ability make neurons work at a slower pace), the micronutrient is scientifically proven to help people stay asleep longer. To get sufficient amounts of magnesium, you'd have to make green leafy veggies a regular part of your diet. If you're the kind of person who doesn't like the taste of vegetables, you could occasionally snack on either almonds or sunflower seeds. Supplementation should be considered as a last resort for one simple reason – pills are often incomplete and inadequate. They're also quite expensive.

You also need to get enough potassium. Much like magnesium, that mineral has sleep-enhancing effects.What makes it stand out though, is its sheer effectiveness in lowering blood pressure. Given that insomnia tends to cause hypertension, potassium's role in blood-pressure regulation isn't something that you should ignore. Tomato sauce (fresh tomatoes are an inferior choice in this case), yogurt (it'd be fine even if you choose the non-fat variant), and sweet potatoes (it doesn't matter how they're prepared, so you can be as creative as you want) all contain considerable amounts ofpotassium.

Melatonin is a Proven Sleep Enhancer

Melatonin affects your sleep cycle in a very straightforward way – whenever there's an abundance of it in your body, you'd easily fall asleep. It is also called the 'sleep hormone'.

Since you're having trouble sleeping, there's a chance that your body isn't producing sufficient amounts of melatonin. Note that the older you get, the less capable your body becomes in terms of producing that hormone. Fortunately for you, there's an easy way to raise the melatonin levels inside your body – eat lots of fruits each day.

As you'd expect though, not all fruits have equal amounts of the sleep-inducing hormone. That's why you should specifically look for bananas, oranges, tart cherries, and pineapples. If you have to choose among those four, you should go for the yellow ones. They've been scientifically proven to boost melatonin levels considerably. Bananas in particular are more than capable of almost doubling the amount of melatonin that circulates throughout the body, while pineapples can nearly triple the hormone's levels.

Link between Exercise and Energy

By simply engaging in enough physical activity daily (cleaning the house doesn't count, at the very least you need to walk around the neighborhood for 30 minutes), you'd be able to keep your energy levels under control.

Exercise makes your body much more capable of tapping into its energy stores during the day, while keeping your nighttime liveliness to a minimum (in a good way, you won't feel extremely groggy or exhausted). In other words, workout routines could actually be considered the key to much more fulfilling days and nights.

Completing the Ultimate Insomnia Cure

Now that you have an in-depth knowledge of the HCCH cure's every aspect, you're more than capable of defeating the most common sleeping disorder and finally get a good sleep. However, it's best to remind you that the cure is designed to be a holistic, encompassing solution – meaning that you'd only get the most out of it, if you don't skip any of its four key parts.

Chapter 22: How To Sleep Better

Most people who are reading this book are going to want to know about the actions that they can take in order to find a deeper and more satisfying sleep at night. There are many simple things that a person can do in order to get a good night's sleep and here are a few of them.Many sleep disorders that we have already discussed may need the help of a physician in order to make sure that your health is maintained. A chronic fatigue is a symptom of a more significant physical issue and needs to be addressed but if you are simply not sleeping as soundly and consistently as you would like there are some simple do's and don'ts that will help you recapture the night.

One of the first things that a person needs to do is to start to keep track of the sleeping patterns that they are experiencing each day. This is easily accomplished by starting a sleep journal.This will be a record that can help a person identify their sleep patterns and the sleeping disorders that they might be suffering from and how to fight it.Keep this handy notebook right next to your bed and keep it diligently each day.

The first data that should be collected for the journal is going to be the times that you go to bed and the time that you wake up each day. Do not record the times before hand, write it down in the morning after you have gotten up for the day.Then make a note of the total hours of sleep that you experienced that night, 8 hours, 6 hours etc.Underneath each basic entry then it is a place for a recap of the sleeping experience. If you had trouble sleeping describe what you did or were thinking about before your fell asleep.Examples would be, closed eyes and thought about work or had a glass of milk, listened to a recorded book.

One of the most important aspects of the sleep journal is to make sure to note all of the food that you had eaten prior to going to bed and the time that you consumed it. This is not a diet journal so there is no need to deceive yourself. Keeping an accurate record of the foods eaten and the times may hold a vital piece of evidence that will help solve your sleeping problem.Along with the food, it is important to record what your feelings and moods were are you headed to bed that night. These can be just as illuminate as the foods that you eat when it comes time to find the cause of your sleeping problem.Finally there should be a strict record kept about any drugs or alcohol that was consumed and the timing of that use.

All of this information will allow you to combine and create a picture of the sleeping patterns that exist in your life and all of the factors that might be affecting you.The sleep journal will allow you to analyze your behavior more objectively and to see if patterns are emerging as you struggle for sleep each night. If eating at a certain time makes your stay awake or if the feelings that you are experience before sleep have a negative or positive effect on you. Making changes can come once you recognize the problems that exist. Identifying your problems and being honest about them is the first step to finding peaceful, restful and rejuvenating sleep each night.

Once all of your information has been gathered then it is time to look at what else can be done in order to help ourselves sleep on a consistent basis and there are many simple things to do in order to achieve this.As human beings we are by nature creatures of habit. It is important to establish consistent sleep routines so that our bodies and our minds become used to this daily rebooting of our systems.Go to sleep and get up at the same time each and every day even on the weekends.If you are varying the time you go to sleep each day, it isn't a wonder that your body doesn't know when it is time to perform or shut down.

The next suggestion is common sense but many people simply ignore it because they feel like they have to. Allow time each day to get the sleep that your require to be rested and perform at your best each day. This can be a major life change for some people. It is important to realize that you deserve to be treated well. Whatever you are doing it is not more important than your health because once your health is gone then so are you. All of the work that seemed so important won't seem so important at the end of your life. Sleep needs to be a priority for your health.

As we discussed before, make sure that it is dark, cool and comfortable where you sleep. This will eliminate distractions and lead you to finding a comfortable and sound night's sleep. This can be a simple lifestyle change, if you realize from your journal that the it is too hot in your room then lower the temperature. You can also move your bed from one area of the room to another, which might provide better lighting or noise protection. These are simple life changes that can bring sound sleep back into your life today.

Shut down the power. There is a common belief that having smart phones, computer tablets or even watching television in bed can harm your sleeping patterns. Many experts advise removing the television from the bedroom because it adds nothing to your sleeping patterns. The associations that we make with a location can cause us to perform to those expectations. If you watch television in bed then your mind might associate bed with entertainment and not bring sound sleep to you.

The smart phone is a creature that is new to sleep problems. Tuning it off at night is a challenge for many people simply can't handle. On the physical level it is believed that the lights from the screen or even the electrical pulse the phone produces can be unhealthy for people and definitely detrimental to great sleeping habits. On the mental level our minds have become so attached to the gaining of information the turning the phone off at night creates anxiety that can take away from sleep.In effect, people are so worried about missing a staus update or a Tweet that they leave their phone on all night long. The fear of cutting this tether of information can cause an anxiety and sleeping disorder all of its own. This type of lifestyle change can be hard but being able to cut the cord of technology to sleep is a great idea. If someone needs to get in touch with you it will wait until morning.

One of the things that you should not do is to treat your insomnia with sleeping pills. For a short time, under a doctor's care the use of drugs for sleeping problems could be acceptable but for the long term a person shouldn't take a sleeping pill to get a good night's sleep. When you take drugs to provide sleep a person is most often addressing the symptom of the problem and not the problem itself. As we discussed before, an inability to sleep is often a symptom of anxiety, depression or a physical ailment that needs to be addressed.In the short term for one night, a sleeping pill might be ok but make sure that they are never taken with alcohol, because this combination can be deadly.

In the end it is important to make sure that our sleep is valued as much as our physical activity or any other aspect of our life. Take the time to learn how to get a good night's sleep and you will be rewarded with a higher quality of life.

Chapter 23:Sleep Hygiene

No matter what kind of day you've had; regardless of the challenges you've struggled with, bed time should become a ritual that signals your brain and body that the time has come to leave it all outside the door of your sleep sanctuary.

While we're often tempted to throw ourselves on the bed with no preparation of our bodies, or the place we're about to lay them for our night's rest, these habits don't serve us. Not engaging in a regular sleep hygiene regimen could be part of the reason we're not sleeping well.

Sleep hygiene forms a barrier between the world we move around in during the day and sleep. It forms a kind of psychological barrier between busyness and rest, and that can prove to be a strong support for improved sleep.

Here are a few of the boxes you need to check off to practice sound sleep hygiene:

• **Go to bed at the same time each night.** Get up at the same time each day. Establishing a sleeping pattern is a cornerstone of getting quality sleep.

• **Avoid stimulants in the evening.** Smoking cigarettes, as well as drinking alcohol and caffeine are habits to avoid in the hours before your appointed bedtime. The alcohol prohibition may seem counter-intuitive, but as your body assimilates alcohol, your sleep may be disrupted, later in the night.

• **Avoid eating after 8 pm.** This practice will also help you maintain you weight, or lose some you may have been wanting to.

Ritual is Restful

At an appointed hour each night, time should be set aside to physically prepare yourself for bed. By performing these self-care rituals each night, you are honoring your sleep time and giving it the prominence in your life it deserves.

Slow Down

Resist the temptation to engage in petty squabbles with loved ones or friends. Let your phone take a message. Don't check your email. It can all wait until tomorrow. Now might be the right time to take a few moments to write in your journal, or do the breathing exercises you've made a part of your daily life.

Your Very Own Turndown Service

Turn down your bed as you might expect it to be, were you staying in a fine hotel.

Light a candle or two. If you've taken to spraying a relaxing scent on your bedclothes, do it now. Arrange your pillows the way you like them to be when you climb into bed.

Dress for Sleep Success

Remove your daytime clothing and put it away (as discussed earlier). If it needs to be washed, make sure it goes in the laundry basket. Change into clean sleeping attire in which you're comfortable and which is dedicated for wear *only* while you're sleeping.

Did You Brush Your Teeth?

I certainly hope so! I hope you also washed your face and brushed or combed your hair. Perhaps a soak in the tub, or a relaxing shower (depending on what works for you). Feeling that you've washed the day off has a finality to it that is another signal it's time to sleep.

It doesn't matter what order you perform these simple rituals in. Performing them as a prelude to sleeping is an effective way of letting your brain know that it's time. Setting aside the time to care for yourself before sleep will help you get the rest you need.

The Big "S"

Who admits to snoring? Almost everyone I know claims they don't snore. I used to, too. Then I woke myself up in mid-snore and all bets were off.

Snoring is a very common problem (so most of us are lying). It has broken up marriages and friendships, kept soldiers awake in barracks and students, in dormitories. It's estimated that almost half the population of the world snores. Of that percentage, 25% are regular sawers of logs. And this tendency is not, by any means, restricted to men! 20% of women snore, too!

But there is so much help now for this unfortunate condition that denial is only cheating those of us who snore out of a decent night's sleep.

Here are a few things you can do to reduce the likelihood of sawing logs that most of us would prefer not to hear sawed in the middle of the night:

● Don't sleep on your back. This sleeping position promotes snoring.

● Try not to smoke cigarettes (or at least, cut down).

● Reduce your alcohol intake.

• Try to lose a little weight (if you need to).

If you're already trying, or have tried employing these strategies and find they aren't helping, visit your General Practitioner to find out what else you might be doing.

There are so many ways to address this noisy (and annoying) problem and new therapies for snoring are being developed every day. In extreme cases, surgery may even be indicated. While that may sound drastic, eliminating this problem will pay off in sound sleep for you and those around you.

Check out the Resources section at the end of this book for some useful information on therapies and devices that can put an end to or reduce habitual snoring.

Conclusion

Thank you again for downloading this book!

I hope this book was able to help you to understand what sleep apnea is and learn about its many available treatments and management steps.

The next step is to loan this book to a loved one with Sleep Apnea to help them use the included tips to rid them of their symptoms and to cure them of Sleep Apnea for good or if you are experiencing it yourself you can use the strategies before complications arise.

Thank you and good luck